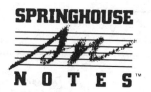

SPRINGHOUSE

N O T E S ™

FLUIDS AND ELECTROLYTES

=== SECOND EDITION ===

Sheryl A. Innerarity, RNC, PhD
Assistant Professor, School of Nursing
University of Texas
Austin
Director of Clinical Nursing
Brackenridge Hospital
Austin

June L. Stark, RN, BSN, MEd
Associate Director of Critical Care Education
New England Medical Center
Boston

Springhouse Corporation
Springhouse, Pennsylvania

Staff

Executive Director, Editorial
Stanley Loeb

Senior Publisher, Trade and Textbooks
Minnie B. Rose, RN, BSN, MEd

Art Director
John Hubbard

Clinical Consultant
Maryann Foley, RN, BSN

Editors
David Moreau, Diane Labus, Nancy Miltenberger

Copy Editors
Diane M. Armento, Pamela Wingrod

Designers
Stephanie Peters (associate art director),
Jacalyn Facciolo

Typography
David Kosten (director), Diane Paluba (manager),
Elizabeth Bergman, Joyce Rossi Biletz, Phyllis
Marron, Robin Mayer, Valerie L. Rosenberger

Manufacturing
Deborah Meiris (director), Anna Brindisi, Kate Davis,
T.A. Landis

Editorial Assistants
Caroline Lemoine, Louise Quinn, Betsy K. Snyder

℞ A member of the Reed Elsevier plc group

Library of Congress Cataloging-in-Publication Data

Innerarity, Sheryl A.
  Fluids and electrolytes/Sheryl A.
Innerarity, June L. Stark. – 2nd ed.
  p. cm. – (Springhouse notes)
  Includes bibliographical references and
index.
  1. Water-electrolyte imbalances – Outlines,
syllabi, etc. 2. Water-electrolyte
imbalances – Nursing – Outlines, syllabi, etc.
3. Water-electrolyte balance (Physiology) –
Outlines, syllabi, etc.
  I. Stark, June L. II. Title. III. Series.
  [DNLM: 1. Acid-Base Equilibrium – outlines.
2. Acid-Base Imbalance – nursing – outlines.
3. Acid-Base Imbalance – outlines.
4. Water-Electrolyte Balance – outlines.
5. Water-Electrolyte Imbalance – outlines.
6. Water-Electrolyte Imbalance – nursing –
outlines. WY 18 I575f 1994]
RC630.I59 1994
616.3'9 – dc20
DNLM/DLC   93-21899
ISBN 0-87434-616-9   CIP

Contents

Advisory Board and Reviewers

REVIEWERS

1st Edition
Luana Martindale, RN, MSN
Associate Professor of Nursing
University of Arkansas, Little Rock

2nd Edition
Linda Carman Copel, PhD, RN, CS
Assistant Professor
College of Nursing
Villanova (Pa.) University

How to Use Springhouse Notes

Springhouse Notes is a multi-volume study guide series developed especially for nursing students. Each volume provides essential course material in an outline format, enabling the student to review the information efficiently.

Special features recur throughout the book to make the information accessible and easy to remember. *Learning objectives* begin each chapter, encouraging the student to evaluate knowledge before and after study. Next, within the outlined text, *key points* are highlighted in shaded blocks to facilitate a quick review of critical information. Key points may include cardinal signs and symptoms, current theories, important steps in a nursing procedure, critical assessment findings, crucial nursing interventions, or successful therapies and treatments. *Points to remember* summarize each chapter's major themes. *Study questions* then offer another opportunity to review material and assess knowledge gained before moving on to new information. Difficult, frequently used, or sometimes misunderstood terms (indicated by small capital letters in the outline) are gathered at the end of each chapter and defined in the *glossary*, Appendix A; answers to the study questions appear in Appendix B.

The Springhouse Notes volumes are designed as learning tools, not as primary information sources. When read conscientiously as a supplement to class attendance and textbook reading, Springhouse Notes can enhance understanding and help improve test scores and final grades.

CHAPTER 1

Essential Concepts of Fluid and Electrolyte Balance

Learning objectives

Check off the following items once you've mastered them:

☐ Describe the characteristics of the homeostatic state.

☐ Identify the fluid, electrolyte, and pH components found in the intracellular and extracellular compartments.

☐ Describe how fluids and electrolytes move between the vascular and interstitial spaces.

☐ State the normal ranges for pH.

I. Introduction

A. Knowledge of the basic concepts of fluid and ELECTROLYTE balance is necessary to provide safe, quality nursing care

B. Fluid and electrolyte balance involves composition and movement of BODY FLUID

C. Body fluids are solutions composed of water and solutes

D. Solutions — liquids (solvents) containing dissolved substances (solutes) — are classified according to their concentration, or *tonicity*, and include the following:
   1. Isotonic solutions *concentration of Electrolytes/non-electrolytes will*
   2. Hypotonic solutions *exert equiv. osmotic pressure of another*
   3. Hypertonic solutions *have higher osmotic pressure*
   Having lower osmotic pressure

E. Body fluids are isotonic solutions

F. Many diseases and disorders can affect fluid and electrolyte balance

G. Solutions ingested into the body through food, drink, or intravenous (I.V.) fluids, as well as fluid lost from the body through vomiting, diarrhea, or excessive perspiration, also can affect fluid and electrolyte balance

II. Homeostasis

A. General information
   1. Homeostasis refers to the state of internal equilibrium within the body when all body systems are in balance
   2. Homeostasis occurs when fluid, electrolyte, and acid-base balance are all maintained within narrow limits despite a wide variation in dietary intake and metabolic rate
   3. Homeostasis is often referred to as a steady state or as equilibrium

B. Key concepts
   1. Water and solutes are distributed throughout the body's compartments
   2. The normal functioning of cells is maintained by the constancy of the body's compartments
   3. To maintain homeostasis, water and solutes are in constant movement and are exchanged continuously
   4. When water and solute concentrations are altered within the body, imbalances develop, disrupting homeostasis

III. Water

A. General information
   1. Body fluid is composed primarily of water
   2. Water is the solvent in which all solutes in the body are either dissolved or suspended

3. For an average-sized man (weight 155 lb [70 kg]), body water accounts for 50% to 60% of total body weight (approximately 40 liters of body water)
4. In women, body water accounts for 45% to 50% of total body weight
5. Women have lower percentages of total body weight as body water than do men because women have a higher percentage of body fat, which does not retain water well
6. In infants, body water represents about 80% of the total body weight
7. In children, the percentage of total weight as body water decreases steadily until it reaches adult percentages by about age 8
8. Obese persons have lower percentages of total weight as body water because adipose tissue does not retain water well

B. Key concepts
1. Body water is contained in two major body compartments, the intracellular fluid (ICF) and the extracellular fluid (ECF)
2. Fluid balance is maintained when water intake equals water output
3. Normally, fluid balance occurs despite wide variations in daily fluid intake
4. The primary source of body fluid intake is water ingestion
5. Water is ingested primarily by drinking fluids and eating foods
6. All foods contain water; almost 100% of the weight of fruit and vegetables and 70% of the weight of meat are water
7. Approximately 350 ml of water are generated daily from digestion and metabolism of carbohydrates, protein, and fat; this is considered intake
8. Under certain circumstances, water can be introduced to the body parenterally (other than through the GI tract) — usually intravenously

IV. Solutes

A. General information
1. Solutes are substances dissolved in a solution
2. Solutes are classified as electrolytes or nonelectrolytes
3. *Nonelectrolytes* are solutes without an electrical charge
4. Nonelectrolytes found in body fluids include glucose, proteins, lipids, oxygen, carbon dioxide, and organic acids
5. *Electrolytes* are solutes that generate an electrical charge when dissolved in water
6. Positively charged electrolytes are called *cations*
7. Major cations in body fluid include sodium (Na), potassium (K), calcium (Ca), magnesium (Mg), and hydrogen (H)
8. Negatively charged electrolytes are called *anions*
9. Major anions in body fluid include chloride (Cl), phosphorus (P), and bicarbonate (HCO_3)

B. Key concepts
   1. The concentration of various solutes in body fluid varies depending on the body fluid compartment
   2. Na is the major cation in the ECF; K is the major cation in the ICF
   3. Electrolytes combine in solutions based on the electrical charge they produce
   4. The chemical combining power of electrolytes is measured in milliequivalent (mEq); 1 mEq of anion reacts chemically with 1 mEq of cation
   5. The total number of cation milliequivalent in body fluids must always equal the total number of anion milliequivalent
   6. Measurement of solute concentration (the number of dissolved particles per liter) in body fluid is based on the fluid's *osmotic pressure,* expressed as either OSMOLALITY or OSMOLARITY
   7. *Osmolality* refers to the number of osmols (the standard unit of osmotic pressure) per kilogram of solution, expressed as milliosmols per kilogram (mOsm/kg)
   8. *Osmolarity* refers to the number of osmols per liter of solution, expressed as mOsm/liter
   9. *Osmolarity* and *osmolality* are commonly used interchangeably; most calculations of body fluid solute concentrations are based on osmolarity

V. Body fluid compartments

A. General information
   1. Body fluid is divided by semipermeable membranes into two major body compartments, the ICF and ECF
   2. The ICF, representing fluid inside the cells, is the largest body compartment
   3. The ICF accounts for about two-thirds of total body fluid
   4. The ECF accounts for about one-third of total body fluid
   5. The ECF is divided into three separate body compartments: interstitial fluid (ISF), intravascular fluid (plasma), and TRANSCELLULAR WATER (TSW)
   6. ISF occupies the spaces between the cells; it constitutes 15% of total body fluid
   7. Plasma is found in the intravascular space and constitutes about 4% of total body fluid or about 75 ml/kg of body weight
   8. TSW constitutes only 1% to 2% of total body fluid and, as such, sometimes is not considered a separate compartment
   9. TSW is usually found in specialized compartments, such as ocular fluid, cerebrospinal fluid, and synovial fluid, as well as in gastric juices

B. Key concepts
   1. Body fluid is not confined to one defined area or compartment; normal body membranes are permeable to water, which facilitates fluid movement through them
   2. Certain solutes are more abundant in certain body compartments and tend to be limited to this compartment under normal conditions; for example, K is more abundant in the ICF, and Na is more abundant in the ECF
   3. Solute movement from one body fluid compartment to another occurs through various mechanisms, such as active and passive transport
   4. Proteins are solutes usually confined to the plasma that create colloid osmotic pressure in the ECF, affecting fluid and solute movement between the ECF and the ICF

VI. Body fluid movement

A. General information
   1. Constant movement of water and solutes between body fluid compartments maintains homeostasis
   2. Membrane permeability and hydrostatic and osmotic pressures affect water and solute movement
   3. Water and solutes move through active and passive transport mechanisms
   4. *Active transport mechanisms* involve chemical activity and the release of energy
   5. Active transport mechanisms include the sodium-potassium pump
   6. *Passive transport mechanisms* do not involve chemical activity or use of energy
   7. Passive transport mechanisms include osmosis and diffusion

B. Key concepts: water movement
   1. All body water movement occurs through *osmosis*
   2. By osmosis, a solvent moves through a semipermeable membrane from an area of lower solute concentration to one of higher concentration
   3. Water movement and distribution depend on the concentration of solute (primarily Na) within a compartment – the compartment's osmolality
   4. Water responds to changes in osmolality because it moves freely between compartments under osmotic or HYDROSTATIC PRESSURE

C. Key concepts: solute movement
   1. Solute movement occurs through active and passive transport (see *Transport Mechanisms*, page 6)
   2. Solute distribution depends on the concentrations of body fluid compartments
   3. Passive transport of solutes is affected by the electrical potential across cell membranes

TRANSPORT MECHANISMS

PASSIVE TRANSPORT MECHANISMS

In **diffusion,** substances move from an area of higher concentration to an area of lower concentration. Movement continues until the molecules are distributed uniformly.

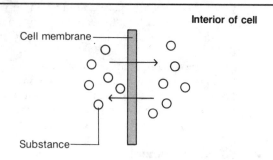

In **osmosis,** water molecules move from an area of higher water concentration (more dilute solution) to an area of lower water concentration (more concentrated solution). The more concentrated solution contains more solute molecules and fewer water molecules; the more dilute solution contains more water molecules and fewer solute molecules.

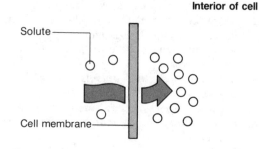

ACTIVE TRANSPORT MECHANISMS

Active transport, a carrier-mediated transport mechanism, moves molecules and ions against a concentration gradient (from lower to higher concentrations). In the **sodium-potassium pump,** active transport moves sodium from inside to outside the cell, where sodium concentration is greater. At the same time, it moves potassium from outside to inside the cell, where potassium concentration is greater.

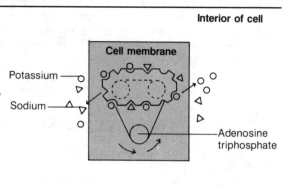

4. By *diffusion,* solutes move from an area of higher solute concentration to one of lower concentration, resulting in an equal distribution of solute
5. *Filtration* requires the force of hydrostatic pressure to move water and some solutes through cell membranes via ultrafication; the fluid produced by this process is known as *ultrafiltrate*
6. Active transport uses an energy source to move solutes from an area of lower solute concentration to one of higher solute concentration against a concentration gradient

D. Key concepts: cellular movement of water and solutes
1. Most solutes move by passive transport mechanisms
2. Active transport, specifically the *sodium-potassium pump,* is necessary to move Na from the cells to the ECF
3. The same pump mechanism drives K from the ECF into the cell; this process allows solutes to move from an area of lower solute concentration to one of higher solute concentration
4. Water moves by osmosis from the ECF to the ICF based on the osmolality of the fluid compartment
5. If the ICF osmolality increases, water will shift from the ECF into the ICF
6. If the ECF osmolality increases, water will shift from the ICF into the ECF

E. Key concepts: vascular movement of water and solutes
1. Movement of water and solutes occurs continuously between the vascular and ISF compartments
2. Movement of water depends on hydrostatic and colloid osmotic pressures in the capillaries; solutes move by diffusion
3. Pressure differences in the venous and arterial ends of capillaries influence the direction and rate of water and solute movement; this process is known as *Starling's law*
4. Colloid osmotic pressures help maintain plasma volume
5. Hydrostatic pressure in the arterial end of the capillary is normally +25 mm Hg, favoring movement of plasma water into the ISF
6. Perivascular tissues exert a pressure of +11 mm Hg, favoring movement of water into the ISF
7. Both forces together exert a pressure of +36 mm Hg, which is opposed by the combined colloidal osmotic pressure of plasma proteins and albumins, a negative pressure of -28 mm Hg
8. The remaining net pressure of +8 mm Hg on the arterial side encourages the movement of water, solutes, and gases from the vascular space to the ISF
9. Hydrostatic pressure in the venous end of the capillary is normally +10 mm Hg (because the venous end is farther from the heart than the arterial end)

10. Interstitial pressure remains +11 mm Hg; the combination of positive venous pressures equals +21 mm Hg, favoring movement of water out of the capillary
11. Plasma proteins exert an opposing pressure of −28 mm Hg, resulting in a total net negative pressure of −7 mm Hg
12. The negative force draws water, metabolic cellular wastes, and carbon dioxide from the ISF into the vascular compartment, resulting in eventual degradation and removal of these substances by a major organ system, such as the lungs or kidneys

VII. Body fluid pH

A. General information
   1. The term *pH* refers to the acidity or alkalinity of a solution, which is determined by the H ion concentration
   2. An H ion donor is considered an ACID
   3. An H ion acceptor is considered a BASE
   4. pH regulation is affected by the dilution of products of metabolism by large volumes of body fluids
   5. All body fluids have a pH; the normal pH of different body fluids varies
   6. The body fluid pH commonly measured to determine acid-base balance is arterial blood pH
   7. Arterial blood pH is regulated through the action of a BUFFER, the lungs, (via K ion exchange), and the kidneys, in that order
   8. The blood pH depends on the HCO_3-carbonic acid ratio in the plasma and ECF

B. Key concepts
   1. Normal arterial blood pH ranges between 7.35 to 7.45
   2. Despite continuous additions of metabolites from cells and food, arterial blood pH usually is maintained at a fairly constant level
   3. An arterial blood pH of ≤6.8 or ≥7.8 is incompatible with life

Points to remember

Homeostasis exists when the intake of fluid and electrolytes equals the output.

Extreme gains or losses of fluids, electrolytes, or acid-base components result in an imbalanced state.

The intracellular fluid (ICF) compartment is composed of fluid within cells; the extracellular fluid compartment (ECF) is composed of the interstitial, intravascular, and transcellular spaces.

Body water and solutes move continuously between the ICF and the ECF.

Body water moves by osmosis; solutes move via passive or active transport mechanisms.

Body fluid pH reflects hydrogen (H) ion concentration.

Glossary

The following terms are defined in Appendix A, page 127.

acid *Substance that is an H ion donor*

base *Substance that is an H ion acceptor*

body fluid *Water + solutes in the ICF + ECF*

buffer *Substance that minimizes pH Δ by adding n absorbing H ions*

electrolyte *elements c̄ an electric charge when in water*

hydrostatic pressure *pressure exerted by a liquid*

osmolality *osmotic pressure measure by milliosmols per kg*

osmolarity *" by milliosmols per liter*

transcellular water *L specialized fluid*

Study questions

To evaluate your understanding of this chapter, answer the following questions in the space provided; then compare your responses with the correct answers in Appendix B, page 130.

1. What type of solution is body fluid? *Isotonic   (=)*
   (Having the same concentration)

2. Into what two major compartments is body water divided? _____
   intracellular (ICF) + Extracellular (ECF)

3. What name is given to solutes that generate an electrical charge when dissolved in water? *electrolytes*

4. What is the major intracellular cation? the major extracellular cation?
   K+   *Na+*

5. What transport mechanism is necessary to move sodium (Na) from the cells to the ECF? *Active transport pump*
   (Na - K+ pump)

6. What is meant by the term pH? *The acidity or alkalinity of a solution*

7. What is the normal arterial blood pH? *7.35 to 7.45*

CHAPTER 2

Water Balance

Learning objectives

Check off the following items once you've mastered them:

☐ State the normal range of serum osmolality.

☐ Describe the relationship between sodium and water balance.

☐ Discuss the process of body water regulation.

☐ Describe the difference between sensible and insensible water losses.

☐ List nursing implications for assessing fluid status.

I. Introduction

A. Water, the most abundant component of body fluid, is required in adequate amounts for body function

B. Water is used by the body to:
1. Act as a solvent for many body chemicals
2. Aid various chemical reactions
3. Maintain stability of body fluids
4. Aid nutrient transport to cells
5. Provide a medium for waste excretion
6. Act as a lubricant between cells to permit friction-free movement
7. Aid body temperature regulation through perspiration
8. Assist in the hydrolysis of food
9. Conduct electrical currents
10. Act as a cushion

C. The body gains and loses water each day; gains and losses must be balanced to maintain body fluid balance (see *Daily Fluid Gains and Losses*)

D. Monitoring fluid intake and output is a valuable tool to determine homeostasis

E. Nursing implications for water balance are as follow:
1. Carefully monitor fluid intake and output
2. When monitoring output, calculate sensible (measurable) losses and estimate insensible losses as closely as possible
3. When it is difficult or impossible to measure urine output, estimate output through other means, such as weighing urine-soaked diapers or incontinence pads, then subtracting the weight of a dry diaper or pad, and converting the weight of urine to a volume measurement
4. For a patient with watery diarrhea, estimate fluid loss by using a bedside commode, bedpan, or other collection device
5. Obtain hourly output measurements, if necessary, to identify a pattern of urine output
6. Monitor for ANURIA, OLIGURIA, or POLYURIA, which would signal serious problems requiring medical intervention
7. Remember that daily weight is an accurate measure of fluid balance; use a history of a patient's weight gain or loss to assess fluid, sodium, and caloric intake
8. To ensure accuracy, weigh the patient daily, using the same scale, before breakfast and when the patient has an empty bladder
9. Correlate daily weight with the 24-hour intake and output, with +500 ml equaling a 1-lb weight gain and −500 ml equaling a 1-lb weight loss
10. Document use of all medications, both over-the-counter and prescription, to anticipate potential fluid-related complications

DAILY FLUID GAINS AND LOSSES

In a healthy person, the fluids ingested balance the fluids excreted (see illustration below). Water loss via the skin and lungs will increase in a hot, dry environment or with increased respiratory rate, fever, or skin injury, such as burns. Water loss via the kidneys varies largely with the amount of solute excreted and with the level of antidiuretic hormone, which controls the kidneys' reabsorption of water.

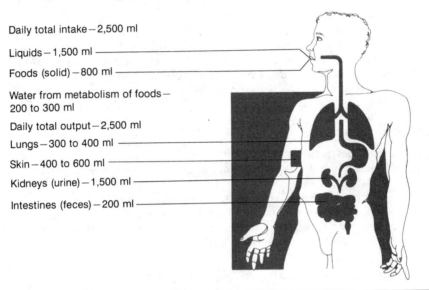

Daily total intake—2,500 ml

Liquids—1,500 ml

Foods (solid)—800 ml

Water from metabolism of foods—
200 to 300 ml

Daily total output—2,500 ml

Lungs—300 to 400 ml

Skin—400 to 600 ml

Kidneys (urine)—1,500 ml

Intestines (feces)—200 ml

11. Monitor urine SPECIFIC GRAVITY and color; if specific gravity is less than or equal to 1.010 and light-colored, diluted urine may indicate overhydration; if specific gravity is greater than or equal to 1.030 and dark-colored, concentrated urine may point to dehydration
12. Remember that a falsely elevated or depressed specific gravity may occur after radiopaque dyes or diuretics are administered, respectively
13. Be aware that specific gravity is not reliable if the patient has renal disease associated with a concentration defect
14. Monitor specific diagnostic tests, such as serum and urine osmolality, blood urea nitrogen, hematocrit, and creatinine, to evaluate water balance

II. Water intake

A. General information
   1. Water must be supplied regularly for metabolic use and to compensate for fluid losses
   2. The total daily intake of water is approximately 2,500 ml

3. The primary source of water is ingested liquids, which account for approximately 1,500 ml/day
4. Water also is obtained by ingesting solid foods, which account for approximately 800 ml/day
5. Food oxidation provides an additional source of water intake, accounting for approximately 200 to 300 ml/day
6. If water cannot be ingested orally, it may be given intravenously

B. Control mechanisms
  1. Water intake is regulated primarily by the thirst sensation
  2. Thirst is stimulated by local responses, such as dry mouth, and systemic responses, such as the action of antidiuretic hormone (ADH), the sensation of a decrease in fluid volume, or an increase in extracellular fluid (ECF) osmolality
  3. Water intake also depends on access to water and the ability to drink

III. Water regulation

A. General information
  1. Water regulation helps maintain a serum osmolality of 280 to 295 mOsm/liter
  2. Water regulation is always associated with sodium regulation
  3. Water balance is regulated by the kidneys, the adrenal cortex, the thirst mechanism, and the secretion or inhibition of ADH; see Chapter 3, Section II, for more information

B. Control mechanisms
  1. Thirst alerts the body to a fluid deficit
  2. The center for thirst control is located in the anterior hypothalamus
  3. OSMORECEPTOR CELLS in the hypothalamus detect a disturbance between the blood plasma and the solutes in the plasma; they sense changes in serum osmolality and initiate impulses to produce the thirst sensation and the release of ADH
  4. Hormonal control of extracellular osmolality is provided by the release or inhibition of ADH, which is produced by the hypothalamus and stored in the posterior pituitary gland
  5. Normal serum osmolality inhibits ADH release, which allows water excretion in the renal tubules
  6. Increased serum osmolality stimulates ADH release, which promotes water reabsorption by the kidneys

IV. Water conservation

A. General information
  1. The body can conserve water when intake does not equal output
  2. The mechanisms that regulate water balance also can conserve water under adverse conditions

B. Control mechanisms
   1. INTRACELLULAR DEHYDRATION stimulates the osmoreceptor cells of the hypothalamus to initiate the thirst sensation
   2. EXTRACELLULAR DEHYDRATION, increased serum osmolality, or a decrease in circulating blood volume also stimulates the hypothalamus to initiate the thirst sensation
   3. An increase in serum osmolality of 1% to 2% (which indicates a water deficit) causes increased secretion of ADH from the posterior pituitary gland to promote water reabsorption in the renal tubules; thus, less urine is excreted
   4. A decrease in circulating blood volume stimulates the cardiac atrial receptors, which, in turn, promote ADH release, leading to increases in water reabsorption by the kidneys and circulating blood volume
   5. Angiotensin II, an end product of renin activation, stimulates secretion of ALDOSTERONE from the adrenal cortex
   6. Aldosterone secretion is regulated by a decrease in circulating blood volume and results in sodium reabsorption by the kidneys
   7. Because sodium and water are closely related, this sodium reabsorption also results in water reabsorption

V. Water excretion

A. General information
   1. Water is excreted through the kidneys, skin, lungs, and gastrointestinal (GI) tract; losses can be categorized as sensible or insensible
   2. Sensible losses are through urine; insensible losses include water lost through the skin, respiratory system, and GI tract
   3. Sensible or insensible losses affect the ECF immediately and, if not replaced, will eventually affect the intracellular fluid

B. Control mechanisms
   1. The kidneys are the major regulatory organs of water balance
   2. Adults lose between 1 and 2 liters of water as urine each day; the amount of urine produced by the kidneys is influenced by ADH and aldosterone levels, and averages approximately 1,500 ml/day
   3. Urine excretion should equal about 1 ml per kilogram of body weight per hour in any age-group
   4. The kidneys have the ability to produce urine with a wide range in osmolality; the range of normal specific gravity is 1.003 to 1.030
   5. The kidneys can excrete urine with a range in osmolality of 200 to 1,400 mOsm/liter without a change in the amount of metabolic wastes or solutes filtered by the tubules
   6. Water loss through perspiration can approach 600 ml/day
   7. The lungs may eliminate 300 to 400 ml of water daily through respiration; increased respiratory rate and depth increase water losses
   8. About 200 ml of water are excreted in feces daily; such water losses may be much greater during GI illness

Points to remember

Water is the main component of body fluid.

Water balance and sodium balance are closely related.

Water balance and sodium balance are regulated by the kidneys, the adrenal cortex, antidiuretic hormone (ADH), aldosterone, and the thirst mechanism.

Monitoring body weight is the most accurate method of assessing fluid status.

The volume and concentration of the urine usually reflect the body's water balance.

Intake and output records provide an estimate of the 24-hour fluid balance.

Glossary

The following terms are defined in Appendix A, page 127.

aldosterone *Hormone that Regulates Na or K Balance*

anuria *No urine output*

extracellular dehydration *Water deficit in the EC compartment*

intracellular dehydration *Water deficit in the IC compartment*

oliguria *daily output of between 50 – 400 mls*

osmoreceptor cells *Specialized cells in hypothalamus that regulate thirst*

polyuria *↑ output (greater than input)*

specific gravity *Weight of a substance in relation to H₂O*

Study questions

To evaluate your understanding of this chapter, answer the following questions in the space provided; then compare your responses with the correct answers in Appendix B, page 130.

1. When a patient's fluid status is assessed, a 1-lb weight gain is equivalent to what amount of fluid gain in milliliters? _____

   500 m/s

2. What is the primary source of water intake? *Ingested liquids*

3. What is the normal range for serum osmolality? _____

   280 - 295 osm/liter

4. What results when serum osmolality increases? *(from pituitary) ADH is released which promotes H2O reabsorption by kidneys (less urine)*

5. What hormones influence the amount of urine produced by the kidneys?

   — Aldosterone (Adrenal Cortex) → Na reabsorption

   — ADH (pituitary)

CHAPTER 3

Electrolyte Balance

Learning objectives

Check off the following items once you've mastered them:

☐ Describe the characteristics of an electrolyte.

☐ List the major intracellular and extracellular electrolytes.

☐ State the functions of sodium, potassium, and calcium.

☐ Explain the role that sodium, potassium, and calcium ions play in normal cardiac function.

I. Introduction

A. Electrolytes, electrically charged solutes in body fluids, are necessary to maintain life

B. Electrolytes perform numerous functions, four of which are essential:
1. They promote neuromuscular irritability
2. They maintain body fluid osmolality
3. They regulate acid-base balance
4. They regulate distribution of body fluids among body fluid compartments

C. Electrolyte imbalance — abnormal excess or deficit of an electrolyte in body fluids — can cause illness

D. Nurses must be aware of the normal functions and levels of electrolytes in the body to better assess and monitor fluid and electrolyte balance in patients

E. Nursing implications for assessing electrolyte balance include the following:
1. Assess overall fluid balance by monitoring daily weight, fluid intake and output, and urine specific gravity; fluid balance is closely related to electrolyte balance; see Appendix C: Fluid Balance Checklist
2. Assess neurologic status, specifically for altered level of consciousness, which may result from an electrolyte imbalance
3. Evaluate motor and sensory function, especially deep tendon reflexes; neuromuscular irritability may indicate electrolyte imbalances
4. Monitor vital signs, especially pulse and blood pressure; certain electrolytes, such as sodium (Na), potassium (K), and magnesium (Mg), directly affect pulse and blood pressure regulation
5. Compare ongoing electrocardiogram (ECG) readings with the patient's baseline ECG to detect changes that may indicate an imbalance
6. Assess respiratory status for changes in rate, depth, and character
7. Monitor serum electrolyte levels for abnormalities (see *Normal Electrolyte Concentration Levels in Intracellular and Extracellular Fluid*, page 20)
8. Remember that electrolytes may be obtained through food intake; be aware of fluids and foods high in certain electrolytes; for more information about food sources, see Appendix D, Food and Fluid Sources of Major Electrolytes
9. Assess nutritional status by monitoring dietary intake and weight; obtain anthropometric measurements and compare with standards
10. Evaluate the patient's health history for medical conditions that might alter electrolyte balance
11. Evaluate the patient's medication history for prescription and over-the-counter drugs that could interfere with electrolyte balance, such as diuretics, antacids, laxatives, and salt substitutes

NORMAL ELECTROLYTE CONCENTRATION LEVELS IN INTRACELLULAR AND EXTRACELLULAR FLUID

Blood contains both intracellular fluid (blood in red blood cells) and extracellular fluid (plasma fluid). Because their cells allow different substances to permeate, intracellular and extracellular fluids have different electrolyte concentration levels. Be aware that standards for these values vary among institutions. *Note:* In the clinical setting, the nurse will see values reflecting the components of extracellular fluid only.

ELECTROLYTE	INTRACELLULAR CONCENTRATION	EXTRACELLULAR CONCENTRATION
Sodium E	10 mEq/liter	135 to 146 m Eq/liter
Potassium I	140 mEq/liter	3.5 to 5.5 mEq/liter
Calcium I	10 mEq/liter	4.0 to 5.5 mEq/liter
Magnesium I	40 mEq/liter	1.5 to 2.5 mEq/liter
Chloride E	4 mEq/liter	96 to 106 mEq/liter
Phosphorus I	100 mEq/liter	1 to 1.5 mEq/liter

II. Sodium (Na)

A. General information
  1. Na is the major cation in the extracellular fluid (ECF)
  2. Normal serum Na concentration in the ECF ranges from 135 to 146 mEq/liter
  3. Normal Na concentration in the intracellular fluid (ICF) is 10 mEq/liter
  4. Excretion or absorption of Na usually involves proportionate excretion or absorption of water and chloride (Cl)
  5. Although the minimum daily Na requirement is 2 g, adults in the United States consume an average of 6 g/day

B. Functions
  1. Na maintains appropriate ECF osmolality
  2. Na maintains ECF volume and influences body water distribution (with Cl)
  3. Na affects the concentration, excretion, and absorption of K and Cl
  4. Na combines readily with bicarbonate (HCO_3) and Cl to help regulate acid-base balance
  5. Na aids impulse transmission in nerve and muscle fibers

C. Regulation
  1. The kidneys mainly regulate Na balance, primarily through ALDOSTERONE action; some Na is excreted through the skin in perspiration

2. The kidneys can adjust Na excretion to match Na intake despite great variations in Na intake
3. The Na level in the ECF is controlled by a feedback loop in which aldosterone secretion by the adrenal cortex stimulates the renal tubules to reabsorb Na
4. A change in serum Na level usually reflects a change in total body water balance
5. Increased Na level in the ECF results in decreased aldosterone production, which increases renal Na excretion
6. Increased Na level in the ECF also raises ECF osmolality, which stimulates antidiuretic hormone (ADH) release that increases renal water reabsorption
7. Decreased Na level in the ECF results in increased aldosterone production, which decreases renal Na excretion
8. Decreased Na level in the ECF also lowers ECF osmolality, which inhibits ADH release and increases renal water excretion

III. Potassium (K)

A. General information
1. K is the major cation in the ICF
2. Normal serum K level ranges from 3.5 to 5.5 mEq/liter
3. Cellular K concentration (usually not measured clinically) is 140 to 145 mEq/liter
4. The daily dietary requirement of K is about 40 mEq; the average daily intake is 60 to 100 mEq
5. K is found in saliva, perspiration, and stomach and intestinal secretions

B. Functions
1. K maintains cell electroneutrality and cell osmolality
2. K directly affects cardiac muscle contraction and electrical conductivity
3. K aids neuromuscular transmission of nerve impulses
4. K plays a major role in acid-base balance; any alteration in K balance will result in acid-base imbalance

C. Regulation
1. K must be ingested daily because the body does not conserve it
2. The kidneys eliminate about 80% of ingested K; about 20 to 40 mEq are lost in each liter of urine
3. The remaining K is excreted in feces (the condition of the bowel influences K absorption); 5 to 10 mEq are lost in each liter of GI fluid
4. K and Na have a reciprocal relationship; the feedback mechanism regulating Na excretion is opposite that regulating K excretion
5. Aldosterone secretion leads to renal Na reabsorption and K excretion

6. Because K ions are exchanged for hydrogen (H) ions in acid-base balances, a decrease in K excretion accompanies an increase in H ION excretion; the opposite is also true
7. The serum K level rises in acidosis and falls in alkalosis; thus, fluctuating serum K levels may or may not reflect an absolute increase or decrease in the total body K level

IV. Chloride (Cl)

A. General information
   1. Cl is the major anion in the ECF
   2. Normal serum Cl level ranges from 96 to 106 mEq/liter

B. Functions
   1. Cl (along with Na) maintains serum osmolality
   2. Cl combines with major cations to create important compounds, such as sodium chloride (NaCl), hydrochloric acid (HCl), potassium chloride (KCl), and calcium chloride (CaCl)
   3. Through HCl production, Cl helps maintain acid-base balance

C. Regulation
   1. Cl balance is tied most closely to Na balance
   2. Cl is indirectly affected by aldosterone
   3. Cl and Na levels usually change in direct proportion to one another
   4. Decreased Cl level (most commonly due to GI losses) results in increased HCO_3 level to balance anions and cations in the ECF

V. Calcium (Ca)

A. General information
   1. Ca is the major cation involved in the structure and function of teeth and bones
   2. About 50% of serum Ca exists in ionized form and is chemically active; this amount is measured as serum Ca
   3. The remaining serum Ca is bound to serum proteins, particularly albumin; because any change in serum protein levels affects the total serum Ca level, the albumin level must be considered with the Ca level
   4. Ca and phosphorus (P) have an inverse relationship; increased serum ·Ca level results in decreased serum P level, and decreased serum Ca level results in increased serum P level
   5. The recommended daily dietary Ca intake is 800 to 1,000 mg daily
   6. Normal serum Ca level ranges from 8.5 to 10.5 mEq/dl (4 to 5.5 mEq/liter)
   7. Normal Ca concentration in the ICF is 10 mEq/liter

B. Functions
   1. Ca (along with P) enhances bone strength and durability

2. Ca helps maintain cell membrane structure, function, and membrane permeability
3. Ca affects activation, excitation, and contraction of cardiac and skeletal muscle
4. Ca participates in neurotransmitter release at synapses
5. Ca helps activate specific steps in blood coagulation
6. Ca activates serum complement, a major factor in immune system function

C. Regulation
1. Ca is absorbed in the small intestine in the presence of vitamin D
2. Vitamin D promotes Ca absorption; P inhibits Ca absorption
3. Ca absorption occurs because of 1,25-dihydroxycholecalciferol (1,25 DCH) (calcitriol); 1,25 DCH is activated vitamin D
4. Parathyroid hormone (PTH) promotes Ca transfer from bone to plasma and aids intestinal and renal Ca absorption
5. Decreased Ca level in the ECF directly stimulates PTH release from the parathyroid glands; this releases calcium phosphate ($CaPO_4$) from bone and indirectly activates mechanisms to increase Ca reabsorption and P excretion from the renal tubules and the GI tract
6. Ca transfer from plasma to bone is aided by calcitonin, which directly lowers serum Ca levels
7. Elevated Ca level in the ECF stimulates the thyroid gland to release calcitonin, which inhibits Ca release from bone and reduces PTH production and release, thereby decreasing mobilization, intestinal absorption, and Ca reabsorption by the kidneys
8. Almost 50% of serum Ca is bound to serum albumin; thus, albumin levels must be considered with Ca levels
   a. A decrease in albumin will lower the Ca level
   b. An increase in albumin will raise the Ca level
9. When serum becomes alkaline, more Ca binds to protein; thus, symptoms of hypocalcemia usually occur during alkalosis
10. Acidosis decreases Ca binding so that acute hyperventilation can temporarily lower serum Ca levels
11. Renal excretion of Ca is limited by calcitriol in deficiency states

VI. Phosphorus (P)

A. General information
1. P is a major anion in the ICF
2. About 80% of P exists in bone in combination with Ca (in a 1:2 ratio of P to C)
3. Normal serum P level ranges from 2.5 to 4.5 mEq/dl (1 to 1.5 mEq/liter)
4. Normal P concentration in the ICF is 100 mEq/liter

B. Functions
1. P is an essential component of bones and teeth (with Ca)

  2. P helps maintain cell membrane integrity
  3. P plays a major role in acid-base balance through its action as a urinary BUFFER; 600 to 900 mg are excreted in the urine daily
  4. P plays essential roles in muscle, red blood cell, and neurologic function and in carbohydrate, protein, and fat metabolism
  5. P functions in cellular metabolism to promote energy transfer to cells

C. Regulation
  1. PTH affects P level by influencing renal excretion of P and increasing Ca reabsorption in response to decreased Ca level in the ECF
  2. Mobilization of P from bone is influenced by PTH levels; see Section V-C of this chapter for more information
  3. Ca and P have an inverse relationship

VII. Magnesium (Mg)

A. General information
  1. Mg is a major cation in the ICF, closely related to Ca and P
  2. About 60% of Mg is contained in bone
  3. A normal diet supplies approximately 25 mEq of Mg daily; of this amount, 10 mEq is absorbed through the small bowel, 10 mEq is excreted in urine, and the remainder is excreted in feces
  4. Normal serum Mg level ranges from 1.5 to 2.5 mEq/liter, with 33% bound to protein and the remainder existing as free cations
  5. Normal Mg concentration in the ICF is 40 mEq/liter

B. Functions
  1. Mg activates intracellular enzymes and acts in carbohydrate and protein metabolism
  2. Mg acts on the MYONEURAL JUNCTION, affecting neuromuscular irritability and contractility of cardiac (antiarrhythmic action) and skeletal muscle
  3. Mg affects peripheral vasodilation, resulting in changes in blood pressure and cardiac output
  4. Mg facilitates transport of Na and K across cell membranes
  5. Mg influences intracellular Ca level through its effect on PTH secretion

C. Regulation
  1. Control of Mg is not clearly understood
  2. Factors that influence Ca and K balance seem to act on Mg as well
  3. Signs and symptoms of Mg imbalance—particularly hypomagnesemia— mimic those of Ca imbalance, which may interfere with diagnosis and treatment of Mg imbalance
  4. The kidneys can conserve Mg efficiently, restricting losses to 1 mEq/ day if necessary; however, excessive Mg excretion can result from diuretic use

Points to remember

Sodium (Na) is the major cation in the ECF.

Potassium (K) is the major cation in the ICF.

Renal and hormonal systems are the major regulators of all electrolytes.

Normal ranges of serum electrolyte levels are as follow: Na, 135 to 146 mEq/liter; K, 3.5 to 5.5 mEq/liter; Cl, 96 to 106 mEq/liter; Ca, 4 to 5.5 mEq/liter; P, 1 to 1.5 mEq/liter; and Mg, 1.5 to 2.5 mEq/liter.

Glossary

The following terms are defined in Appendix A, page 127.

aldosterone

buffer

ion

myoneural junction

Study questions

To evaluate your understanding of this chapter, answer the following questions in the space provided; then compare your responses with the correct answers in Appendix B, pages 130 and 131.

1. How is the sodium (Na) level in the extracellular fluid (ECF) controlled?

_____

_____

2. What are two major functions of potassium (K)? _____

_____

_____

3. What is the relationship between Na and K? _____

_____

_____

4. What would the nurse expect to see if a patient experiences decreased chloride (Cl) levels from vomiting? _____

_____

5. When a patient's serum becomes alkaline, what would the nurse expect to see? _____

_____

6. What are three functions of magnesium (Mg)? _____

_____

_____

CHAPTER 4

Acid-Base Balance

Learning objectives

Check off the following items once you've mastered them:

☐ Describe the characteristics of an acid and a base.

☐ State the alterations in pH that occur in acidosis and in alkalosis.

☐ Describe the roles of the renal and respiratory systems in buffering and regulating acid-base balance.

☐ Identify the normal values for an arterial blood gas analysis.

☐ Describe renal and respiratory compensation.

I. Introduction

A. Acid-base balance refers to homeostasis of the hydrogen (H) ion concentration in body fluids

B. Body fluids are classified as acids or bases according to their H ion concentration
   1. An ACID is an H ion donor
   2. A BASE is an H ion acceptor

C. Acid-base balance is maintained by controlling the H ion concentration of body fluids, specifically extracellular fluid (ECF)
   1. The concentration of H ions in a body fluid is expressed as the pH
   2. The numerical value of the pH is inversely proportional to the number of H ions in solution; the pH falls as the H ion concentration rises; the reverse is also true

D. Normal blood pH ranges from 7.35 to 7.45; a pH below 6.8 or above 7.8 is incompatible with life

E. ACIDOSIS defines an excess of H ions as either acid excess or base deficit and is marked by pH less than 7.35

F. ALKALOSIS defines a deficit of H ions as either base excess or acid deficit and is marked by pH more than 7.45

G. A patient's acid-base balance is evaluated by blood gas analysis of either arterial or capillary (children) blood

II. Measurement of acid-base balance

A. General information
   1. Because acids and bases leave the body mainly through gas exchange between the cells and the external environment, measurement of these gases reflects acid-base balance
   2. Blood gas measurements are the major diagnostic tool for evaluating acid-base balance
   3. Commonly used blood gas measurements include arterial blood gas (ABG) and mixed venous blood gas measurements
   4. Related methods of measurement include transcutaneous blood gas measurements, pulse oximetry, serum anion gap measurements, serum potassium (K) levels, and total carbon dioxide (CO_2) and chloride (Cl) levels
   5. ABG levels are analyzed in blood samples obtained from an artery, such as the radial, brachial, or femoral artery, or from an arterial line; mixed venous blood gas levels are analyzed in blood samples taken from a pulmonary artery catheter or a central venous catheter

NORMAL A.B.G. VALUES

The normal values shown below may vary slightly from one laboratory to another, depending on testing methods used. These values apply to adults at sea level.

PARAMETER	NORMAL RANGE
pH	7.35 to 7.45
$PaCO_2$	35 to 45 mm Hg
HCO_3	22 to 26 mEq/liter
Base excess	-2 to $+2$
PaO_2	80 to 100 mm Hg
SaO_2	95% to 100%

B. ABG measurements
1. ABG levels help to determine a patient's acid-base status, evaluate pulmonary gas exchange efficiency, assess the respiratory system, evaluate blood oxygenation, and monitor respiratory therapy (see *Normal ABG Values*)
2. ABG measurements include the following six parameters:
   a. pH
   b. Partial pressure of CO_2 in arterial blood ($PaCO_2$)
   c. Bicarbonate (HCO_3) concentration
   d. Base excess
   e. Partial pressure of oxygen in arterial blood (PaO_2)
   f. Oxygen saturation (O_2 Sat or SaO_2)
3. pH indicates blood acidity; values greater than 7.45 indicate alkalosis, and values less than 7.35 indicate acidosis
4. A normal or borderline pH may indicate a normal acid-base balance or the body's attempts at compensating for a slightly abnormal or chronic acid-base imbalance
5. $PaCO_2$ levels indicate the partial pressure of CO_2 in arterial blood and are used to evaluate the respiratory acid-base component
6. $PaCO_2$ values greater than 45 mm Hg indicate hypoventilation or excessive CO_2 retention (hypercapnia) and, therefore, acidosis; values less than 35 mm Hg indicate hyperventilation or excessive CO_2 exhalation (hypocapnia) and, therefore, alkalosis
7. HCO_3 levels reflect the arterial blood's HCO_3 concentration and are used to evaluate the metabolic acid-base component
8. HCO_3 values greater than 26 mEq/liter indicate alkalosis; values less than 22 mEq/liter indicate acidosis

NORMAL MIXED VENOUS BLOOD GAS VALUES

The normal values shown below may vary slightly from one laboratory to another, de-pending on testing methods used. These values apply to adults at sea level.

PARAMETER	NORMAL RANGE
pH	7.39 to 7.41
$P\bar{v}CO_2$	41 to 51 mm Hg
HCO_3	22 to 26 mEq/liter
Base excess	-2 to +2
$P\bar{v}O_2$	35 to 40 mm Hg
$S\bar{v}O_2$	70% to 75%

9. Base excess reflects the level of HCO_3 and other bases, such as plasma proteins and hemoglobin, and is used to evaluate the metabolic acid-base component
10. Base excess values greater than +2 indicate a base excess (acid deficit) in metabolic alkalosis; values less than −2 indicate a base deficit (acid excess) in metabolic acidosis
11. PaO_2 and SaO_2 levels are secondary parameters in assessing acid-base status
12. PaO_2 levels reflect the partial pressure of oxygen in arterial blood, revealing the lungs' ability to oxygenate blood
13. PaO_2 levels are not used to evaluate acid-base status
14. PaO_2 values less than 80 mm Hg indicate hypoxemia (for each year over age 60, subtract 1 mm Hg from the normal PaO_2 range to determine the normal range for a patient of that age)
15. SaO_2 levels reflect the oxygen-carrying capacity of hemoglobin and help evaluate respiratory function; see Appendix E, Arterial Blood Gas Findings and Interpretations

C. Mixed venous blood gas measurements
   1. Measuring mixed venous blood gases is an increasingly common method of assessing acid-base balance
   2. Mixed venous blood gas measurement reflects the blood gas composition in the alveoli
   3. It also reflects pulmonary capillary ventilation and perfusion
   4. Mixed venous blood gas measurements include the following six parameters:
      a. pH
      b. Partial pressure of CO_2 in mixed venous blood (P-vCO_2)
      c. HCO_3 concentration
      d. Base excess

e. Partial pressure of oxygen in mixed venous blood (P-vO_2)

f. Oxygen saturation in mixed venous blood (S-vO_2)

5. Most mixed venous blood gas measurement values are similar to and correlate well with ABGs if the patient's cardiac output remains relatively constant (see *Normal Mixed Venous Blood Gas Values)*

III. Buffer regulation of acid-base balance

A. General information

1. Despite continuous additions of metabolites from cells and food, body pH is maintained at a fairly constant level; H ion concentration is affected by dilution of products of metabolism by large volumes of water (H_2O)

2. Metabolism produces 50 to 100 ions of H daily and about 15,000 mmole of CO_2 daily

3. The kidneys excrete only 1% of this amount; the lungs and other buffers handle the rest

4. The cells function as buffers by taking up or releasing extra H ions; this process involves exchanging K for H and, thus, affects K balance

5. Buffers regulate H ion concentration by taking up or releasing H or hydroxyl ions

6. Buffers temporarily minimize the effect of H or HCO_3 on blood pH until the renal or respiratory system takes effect

B. Carbonic acid (H_2CO_3) and sodium bicarbonate ($NaHCO_3$) as buffers

1. The major extracellular chemical buffers are H_2CO_3 and $NaHCO_3$

2. These buffers are the first to react to a change in pH, but their effect is relatively brief

3. HCO_3 acts to maintain a ratio of 20 parts HCO_3 to 1 part H_2CO_3, maintaining blood pH at 7.45

4. HCO_3 buffering action is expressed by the equation $CO_2 + H_2O \rightleftharpoons H_2CO_3 \rightleftharpoons H + HCO_3$

5. The lungs retain or eliminate CO_2, increasing or decreasing H_2CO_3 concentration

C. Phosphate buffers

1. Phosphates act as buffers in essentially the same way as the HCO_3-H_2CO_3 system

2. They play an important role in regulating pH in red blood cells and renal tubular fluids

3. Monosodium or potassium phosphates are buffers; concentrations are regulated by the kidneys

D. Protein buffers

1. Protein buffers are the most abundant buffers in body cells and blood

2. Oxyhemoglobin gives up its oxygen to the body cells to become reduced hemoglobin, which combines with H ion levels to form a weak acid and, thereby, act as a buffer

3. Acid proteinate and neutral proteins also function as buffers

IV. Respiratory system regulation and compensation

A. General information
1. The lungs are the first line of protection in acid-base regulation, capable of responding to changes within minutes
2. Alteration in pulmonary function or cessation of respirations usually results in acid-base imbalances

B. Regulation
1. The lungs regulate H ion concentration by eliminating CO_2 (which combines with H_2O to form H_2CO_3
2. Excessive H_2CO_3 is reduced in the lungs to H_2O and CO_2, which is excreted during breathing
3. H_2CO_3 in the alveolar capillaries crosses into the alveoli and is broken down into CO_2 and H_2O, thereby eliminating an H ion; the reverse reaction also occurs
4. This is accomplished by adjusting the rate and depth of ventilation in response to the CO_2 level in the blood ($PaCO_2$)
5. Increased $PaCO_2$ level or low pH results in an increased respiratory rate and *hyperventilation*, causing increased exhalation of CO_2 and thus raising blood pH
6. Decreased $PaCO_2$ level or high pH results in a decreased respiratory rate and *hypoventilation*, causing CO_2 retention and thus lowering blood pH

C. Compensation
1. The lungs can compensate for metabolic disturbances by either retaining or removing CO_2, thus minimizing the change in serum pH
2. HCO_3 excess (metabolic alkalosis) suppresses the rate and depth of respirations, causing CO_2 retention and H_2CO_3 buildup
3. HCO_3 deficit (metabolic acidosis) causes increased rate and depth of respirations and greater elimination of CO_2

V. Renal system regulation and compensation

A. General information
1. The renal system is the slowest of all the regulating systems; it takes from a few hours to several days to adjust to changes
2. The kidneys excrete only 1% of the H ion excess; therefore, they are slow to compensate for acid-base imbalances, usually requiring 24 to 48 hours
3. The renal system, however, can permanently adjust blood pH
4. Normal renal regulation involves the following reactions in the renal tubules:
    a. K secretion
    b. Na and HCO_3 reabsorption into the body

      c. H secretion into the tubules

B. Regulation
1. The kidneys may excrete either acidic or alkaline urine to compensate for excesses, but the urine is usually acid
2. The kidneys reabsorb HCO_3 from the renal tubules in a state of acid excess and excrete HCO_3 in a state of acid deficit
3. H ions combine with phosphates and are excreted as phosphoric acid to conserve Na and K; H ions are removed and HCO_3 is added to the blood
4. The kidneys regulate H ion concentration by combining H with ammonia (NH_3) to form ammonium (NH_4); the reverse reaction is also true
5. In the formation of NH_4, H is removed and HCO_3 is added to the blood
6. NH_4 is excreted when H ions must be eliminated

C. Compensation
1. The kidneys compensate for respiratory imbalances by excreting or retaining H and HCO_3
2. In H_2CO_3 excess, the kidneys excrete H and conserve HCO_3 to restore balance
3. In H_2CO_3 deficit, the kidneys retain H and excrete HCO_3 to restore balance
4. H is exchanged for K to raise or lower the pH

Points to remember

Hydrogen (H) ion content in the body determines pH.

A hydrogen ion excess or a base deficit results in acidosis.

A hydrogen ion deficit or a base excess results in alkalosis.

Normal blood pH ranges from 7.35 to 7.45.

Arterial blood gas (ABG) levels help to determine a patient's acid-base status, evaluate pulmonary gas exchange efficiency, assess the respiratory system, evaluate blood oxygenation, and monitor respiratory therapy.

Glossary

The following terms are defined in Appendix A, page 127.

acid

acidosis

alkalosis

base

Study questions

To evaluate your understanding of this chapter, answer the following questions in the space provided; then compare your responses with the correct answers in Appendix B, page 131.

1. What do partial pressure of CO_2 in arterial blood ($PaCO_2$) values indicate?

_____

_____

2. What is the normal range for bicarbonate (HCO_3) values? _____

_____

_____

3. What are the major extracellular chemical buffers? _____

_____

_____

4. What organs are the first line of protection in acid-base regulation and are capable of responding to changes in minutes? _____

_____

5. How does the body attempt to compensate for metabolic acidosis?

_____

_____

6. How do the kidneys regulate acid-base balance? _____

_____

_____

CHAPTER 5

Water Imbalances

Learning objectives

Check off the following items once you've mastered them:

☐ Describe the difference between isotonic, hypotonic, and hypertonic water imbalances.

☐ List the clinical manifestations of each type of water imbalance.

☐ Discuss nursing implications for each type of water imbalance.

☐ Describe patients at greatest risk for water imbalances.

I. Introduction

A. Imbalances in body fluids are of three common types: ISOTONIC, HYPOTONIC, and HYPERTONIC

B. Imbalances also can be classified as volume or osmotic imbalances
   1. Volume imbalances primarily affect the extracellular fluid (ECF) and involve relatively equal losses or gains of sodium (Na) and water
   2. Osmotic imbalances primarily affect the intracellular fluid (ICF) and involve relatively unequal losses or gains of Na and water

C. Excessive loss of water may result in dehydration

II. ECF volume deficit (isotonic fluid volume deficit)

A. General information
   1. ECF volume deficit results from relatively equal losses of Na and water
   2. Volume losses occur from the ECF, but because the Na to water ratio remains essentially unchanged, osmolality is not affected
   3. Because osmolality is unchanged, regulatory mechanisms – such as antidiuretic hormone (ADH) and aldosterone secretion – are not activated, and fluid ordinarily does not shift from the ICF to the ECF

B. Etiology
   1. Prolonged vomiting or gastric suction
   2. Excessive diarrhea
   3. Hemorrhage
   4. Profound urine loss, such as polyuria from diabetic ketoacidosis or diuresis
   5. Fever
   6. THIRD-SPACE shifting, such as occurs in burns, intestinal obstruction, and peritonitis

C. Clinical manifestations
   1. Weight loss
   2. Hypotension
   3. Orthostatic hypotension
   4. Tachycardia
   5. Oliguria
   6. Decreased skin turgor
   7. Dry, furrowed tongue
   8. Soft eyeballs (can be detected by applying gentle pressure on top of the eyelid)
   9. Sticky oral mucosa
   10. Altered level of consciousness (LOC)
   11. Slow-filling jugular veins

D. Diagnostic findings
   1. Increased urine specific gravity

    2. Increased hematocrit
    3. Increased serum protein level
    4. Increased blood urea nitrogen (BUN) level
    5. Normal serum Na level (usually)
    6. Normal serum creatinine level in relation to an elevated BUN level

E. Nursing implications
    1. Monitor fluid intake and output to determine the need for replacement therapy
    2. Check daily weight to note loss that may indicate fluid deficit (a 1-lb weight loss equals a 500-ml fluid loss)
    3. Monitor vital signs to detect increased pulse or decreased blood pressure
    4. Assess skin turgor by evaluating resilience and resistance on the forehead or the shoulders; easily pinched skin in these locations may indicate volume deficit (the extremities are not as useful for assessing skin turgor because of skin changes that normally occur with aging and disease conditions)
    5. Assess oral mucous membranes; sticky mucous membranes and a dry tongue may indicate fluid volume loss
    6. Monitor the results of laboratory studies—particularly BUN and hematocrit levels, which may increase in volume deficit
    7. Assess LOC; altered LOC may occur in severe volume deficit
    8. Administer fluid replacement as indicated and as ordered; fluid replacement should match the type of loss; intravenous (I.V.) fluids may be indicated for moderate or severe fluid deficits; oral fluids may be indicated for mild deficits
    9. Monitor parenteral fluid administration; when one imbalance is treated, the opposite imbalance may occur as a result of therapy
    10. Provide frequent oral care to prevent breakdown of dry mucous membranes
    11. Turn the patient at least every 2 hours to prevent skin breakdown, a problem of particular concern for a patient with volume deficit

III. ECF volume excess (isotonic fluid volume excess)

A. General information
    1. ECF volume excess, also termed *overhydration,* results from relatively equal gains of Na and water in the ECF
    2. Osmolality is not significantly affected because fluid and solute gains occur in equal proportions
    3. As excessive isotonic fluid accumulates in the ECF, fluid shifts into the interstitial space, resulting in edema

B. Etiology
    1. Iatrogenic overinfusion of parenteral fluids, particularly 0.9% sodium chloride (NaCl)

2. Administration of hypertonic parenteral fluids, such as 3% or 5% NaCl
3. Excessive ingestion of solutes, such as Na, in foods or medications
4. Excessive administration of saline solution enemas
5. Corticosteroid administration
6. Congestive heart failure
7. Chronic renal failure, with accumulation of fluid and solutes between dialysis treatments
8. Chronic liver disease
9. Hypoalbuminemia, which may be associated with renal disease or malnutrition

C. Clinical manifestations
   1. Acute weight gain
   2. Distended neck veins
   3. Polyuria (with normal renal function)
   4. Elevated blood pressure
   5. Full, bounding pulse
   6. Crackles auscultated in lung fields
   7. Dyspnea
   8. Tachypnea
   9. Ascites
  10. Peripheral edema

D. Diagnostic findings
   1. Decreased hematocrit (resulting from hemodilution)
   2. Normal serum Na level
   3. Abnormal chest X-ray indicating fluid accumulation (for example, pulmonary edema or pleural effusions)

E. Nursing implications
   1. Monitor fluid intake and output for indications of excess
   2. Monitor daily weight for increases that may indicate fluid excess; keep in mind that a 1-lb weight gain equals 500-ml of fluid gain
   3. Monitor cardiopulmonary status; assess for increased blood pressure and respiratory rate
   4. Auscultate lung sounds; note crackles that do not clear with coughing, which may indicate fluid retention
   5. Assess for subjective complaints of dyspnea, such as complaints of shortness of breath or exertional dyspnea
   6. Monitor chest X-ray results to detect changes pointing to fluid accumulation
   7. Monitor laboratory study results for decreased BUN and hematocrit levels
   8. Assess for presence and amount of peripheral edema
   9. Inspect the patient confined to bed rest for sacral edema (the sacrum may be the only place that fluid accumulates in the supine position)

10. Make sure that the patient turns at least every 2 hours; edematous skin is more prone to breakdown
11. Monitor infusion of parenteral fluids if ordered; check the rate every hour, and use I.V. controllers (pumps) as necessary to prevent fluid overload
12. Monitor the therapeutic and adverse effects of prescribed medications, especially those that may potentiate the imbalance
13. Teach the patient and family to monitor and record fluid intake and output and daily weight
14. Teach the patient and family about the effects of Na intake on fluid balance and about which food and fluids to avoid
15. Teach the patient and family how to safely administer prescribed medications

IV. ICF volume excess (hypotonic or hypo-osmotic fluid volume excess)

A. General information
1. ICF volume excess results from a disproportionately high loss of Na in relation to water in the ECF
2. Na loss occurs initially from the ECF, leaving the ECF hypotonic; as a result, the cell is hypertonic and fluid will move from the ECF into the ICF to achieve osmotic equilibrium, thereby creating a hypotonic fluid excess in the ICF
3. ICF volume excess also may result from an increase in solute-free fluid in the ECF, for example, from overadministration of dextrose 5% in water
4. ICF volume excess should be considered as hyponatremia because Na is the primary ECF ion and the clinical manifestations are essentially the same
5. Osmotic changes result from a disproportionately low concentration of Na in relation to water; serum osmolality decreases to below 285 mOsm/liter
6. Accumulation of hypo-osmotic fluid in the ICF results in a "central" intracellular edema
7. Intracellular edema causes increased intracranial pressure, which produces the primary signs and symptoms related to the central nervous system (CNS), such as confusion and disorientation

B. Etiology
1. Prolonged diuretic therapy with low salt intake
2. Replacement of lost body fluids (as from severe diaphoresis or hemorrhage) with only water or other Na-free fluids
3. Excessive water intake linked to psychological disturbance
4. Nasogastric (NG) tube irrigation with tap water
5. Excessive amounts of ice chips given to patients with NG tubes or to patients who are vomiting

6. Excessive release of ADH caused by stress, surgery, trauma, or narcotic use
7. Excessive I.V. administration of hypotonic fluids
8. Excessive administration of tap water enemas
9. Congestive heart failure
10. Oat cell carcinoma of the lung, which may be associated with syndrome of inappropriate ADH (SIADH) secretion
11. Prolonged use of oral hypoglycemic agents
12. Prolonged use of tricyclic antidepressants
13. Alcoholism

C. Clinical manifestations
1. Confusion and disorientation
2. Muscle twitching
3. Hyperirritability
4. Mental disturbances, such as personality changes
5. Headache
6. Nausea and vomiting
7. Convulsions
8. Coma
9. Polyuria in patients with healthy kidneys

D. Diagnostic findings
1. Serum Na level less than 120 mEq/liter
2. Serum osmolality less than 285 mOsm/liter
3. Hypoproteinemia

E. Nursing implications
1. Monitor intake and output for indications of fluid excess
2. Obtain daily weight to assess for fluid excess; remember that a 1-lb weight gain equals a 500-ml fluid gain (approximately 1 kg of weight gain equals 1 liter of fluid gain)
3. Monitor vital signs for changes pointing to fluid excess
4. Assess LOC and mental status for changes in cognitive function, orientation, or personality
5. Restrict fluids as ordered
6. If parenteral fluid administration is ordered, monitor infusion carefully to ensure a patent I.V. line and an accurate infusion rate
7. Administer hypotonic parenteral fluid carefully; changes in output related to weight and correlated with CNS manifestations may prevent the development of hypo-osmotic conditions
8. Monitor laboratory study results for decreasing serum Na level and serum osmolality

V. ICF volume deficit (hypertonic or hyperosmotic fluid volume deficit)

A. General information
   1. ICF volume deficit results from a disproportionately high loss of water in relation to Na in the ECF
   2. Excessive water loss from the ECF leaves the ECF hypertonic; as a result, water moves from the ICF into the ECF, creating a hypertonic fluid deficit in the ICF
   3. ICF volume deficit should be considered hypernatremia because Na is the primary ion affected
   4. The osmolality of the ICF and the ECF eventually reaches an equilibrium, creating hypertonicity of both compartments when water has been lost without a corresponding solute loss
   5. Serum osmolality increases because of this hypertonicity

B. Etiology
   1. Excessive insensible water losses, as from tachypnea, hyperventilation, hyperthermia, or severe diaphoresis
   2. Decreased water intake, as from dysphagia, debilitating conditions, stroke, or coma
   3. Prolonged nothing-by-mouth (NPO) status without adequate parenteral fluid replacement
   4. Excessive administration of hypertonic fluids
   5. Excessive administration of sodium bicarbonate to treat metabolic acidosis
   6. Administration of tube feedings inadequately diluted with water
   7. Prolonged total parenteral nutrition therapy
   8. Hyperglycemia
   9. Severe gastroenteritis or diarrhea

C. Clinical manifestations
   1. Weakness
   2. Restlessness
   3. Delirium
   4. Tetany
   5. Hyperventilation
   6. Thirst
   7. Irritability
   8. Fever
   9. Flushed skin
   10. Oliguria
   11. Hyperactive deep tendon reflexes
   12. Grand mal seizures
   13. Sudden respiratory arrest

D. Diagnostic findings
   1. Serum Na level greater than 145 mEq/liter

   2. Serum osmolality greater than 300 mOsm/liter
   3. Moderately high to normal hematocrit
   4. Urine specific gravity greater than 1.030

E. Nursing implications
   1. To restore osmolality and lower serum Na levels, administer fluids as ordered—usually hypotonic I.V. fluids through a volume control device
   2. Monitor fluid intake and output for decreased output
   3. Obtain daily weight to distinguish weight loss from fluid loss
   4. Monitor LOC for changes that may result from too rapid infusion of hypotonic fluid
   5. Monitor serum Na level and serum osmolality
   6. Assess patients who are NPO for surgery or diagnostic studies for signs and symptoms of water loss
   7. Dilute tube feedings with adequate amounts of water to prevent administration of hypertonic fluids

VI. Third-space fluid shifting

A. General information
   1. *Third-space fluid shifting* describes fluid accumulation in an abnormal compartment (one other than the ECF or the ICF)
   2. Creation of a "third space" requires a cellular membrane that allows water and fluid to enter but not to exit
   3. Water and electrolytes in a third space are not available to maintain normal body fluid compartments; solute and water imbalances result
   4. Accumulation of third-space fluids usually involves swelling from inflammation with concurrent loss of fluids
   5. Some third-space fluids result from osmotic changes caused by loss of protein—for example, ascites associated with urinary protein loss
   6. Third-space fluid eventually may be reabsorbed or must be removed mechanically by procedures such as paracentesis or thoracentesis

B. Etiology
   1. Acute bowel obstruction
   2. Ascites
   3. Hypoalbuminemia
   4. Pleural effusion
   5. Acute peritonitis
   6. Burns
   7. Pancreatitis

C. Clinical manifestations
   1. Hyponatremia
   2. Tachycardia
   3. Hypotension
   4. Oliguria, with urine output less than 30 ml/hour
   5. Low central venous pressure

6. Poor skin and tongue turgor
7. Weight changes (usually gains)

D. Diagnostic findings
   1. Elevated urine specific gravity
   2. Elevated serum hematocrit

E. Nursing implications
   1. Keep in mind that third-space fluid shifting is an acute and serious problem
   2. Monitor and document the following to assess the extent and severity of the third-space shift: pulse rate and rhythm, blood pressure, respiratory rate, fluid intake and output, daily weight, abdominal girth, and urine specific gravity and osmolality
   3. Remember that monitoring these values will also assist in estimating fluid movement changes from the third space back to normal fluid compartments
   4. Keep in mind that parenteral fluid administration will provide symptomatic relief but will not resolve the problem; rather, it will increase the patient's total body weight without making the third-space fluid available to the body
   5. Be aware that correction may require surgery, such as the insertion of a peritonvenous shunt, or correction may occur spontaneously as a physiologic shift that can be predicted to occur within 48 to 72 hours

VII. Patients at risk for water imbalances

A. General information
   1. Certain disease states, medication use, and age are factors influencing a person's susceptibility to water imbalances
   2. These factors affect the routes of water gains or losses, homeostatic regulatory systems, or the body's ability to compensate for imbalances
   3. The three groups of patients most at risk are as follow:
      a. Infants and children because of the immaturity of their regulatory mechanisms and physiologic differences in body composition
      b. Older adults because of physiologic changes, decreased access from compromised mobility, and diminished compensatory reserves
      c. Chronically ill patients because of increased physiologic stress and diminished compensatory reserves

B. Newborns, infants, and children
   1. In newborns, water constitutes 80% of total body weight (90% in premature newborns)
   2. In infants, about 40% of body water is in the ECF, compared with 20% in adults
   3. By age 2, a child's percentage of total body weight as water approaches 50%, as in an adult

4. An infant may exchange 50% of the ECF daily, compared with 18% in an adult
5. The immature kidneys concentrate urine inefficiently and, combined with the previous factors, contribute to the potential for rapid dehydration in disease states
6. Compared with adults who may be able to tolerate fluid imbalances for days, infants and young children can develop an acute imbalance in hours
7. Because the ratio of body surface area to weight is several times greater in infants and children than in adults, infants and children are at greater risk for fluid imbalance from insensible water loss through the skin
8. Because infants and children have a relatively greater gastrointestinal tract surface area, they can experience greater water losses there

C. Older adults
1. After age 65, the percentage of total body water progressively decreases to between 40% and 50%
2. Progressively decreasing renal function impairs excretion of heavy solute loads, such as those from tube feedings
3. Risk of hyperglycemia and osmotic diuresis increases because of decreased pancreatic functioning and glucose tolerance
4. Cardiovascular function deterioration impairs compensation for hypotensive states
5. Decreased mobility and cognition may compromise consumption of adequate fluids (and foods), particularly during illness
6. Diminished thirst mechanism increases the risk of dehydration, especially in hot weather
7. Diminished renal function increases the risk of water imbalance from certain medications, particularly diuretics and electrolyte replacement supplements
8. Decreased skin elasticity makes skin turgor a poor indicator of hydration status

D. Chronically ill patients
1. Illness affecting major body systems may compromise changes in fluid balance
2. Diabetes and other endocrine diseases indirectly affect fluid balance
3. Patients with renal insufficiency or chronic renal failure must maintain proper fluid balance to prevent acute illness

Points to remember

Isotonic imbalances primarily affect the extracellular fluid (ECF) and involve relatively equal losses or gains of sodium (Na) and water.

Hypotonic and hypertonic imbalances primarily affect the intracellular fluid (ICF) and involve relatively unequal losses or gains of sodium (Na) and water.

Edema results from the accumulation of fluid in the interstitial space.

Third-space shifting involves fluid accumulation in an abnormal compartment, one other than the ECF or the ICF, such as the peritoneal cavity.

Those at greatest risk for water imbalances are infants and children, older adults, and chronically ill patients.

Glossary

The following terms are defined in Appendix A, page 127.

hypertonic

hypotonic

isotonic

third space

Study questions

To evaluate your understanding of this chapter, answer the following questions in the space provided; then compare your responses with the correct answers in Appendix B, pages 131 and 132.

1. What substances are lost to result in an ECF volume deficit? _____
_____
_____

2. What are four clinical manifestations in an ECF volume excess?
_____
_____

3. From what does an ICF volume excess result? _____
_____
_____

4. What are three key causes of ICF volume excess? _____
_____
_____

5. When a patient with ICF volume deficit is assessed, what would the patient's serum Na level be? _____
_____

6. What nursing interventions are important for the patient experiencing a third-space fluid shift? _____
_____

CHAPTER 6

Electrolyte Imbalances

Learning objectives

Check off the following items once you've mastered them:

☐ State laboratory test values representative of each electrolyte imbalance.

☐ List the clinical manifestations of each electrolyte imbalance.

☐ Describe the nursing implications for a patient for each electrolyte imbalance.

☐ Identify the ECG changes that occur with potassium, calcium, and magnesium imbalances.

☐ Describe those patients at greatest risk for electrolyte imbalances.

I. Introduction

A. Electrolyte imbalances are common in patients requiring nursing care

B. Certain electrolyte imbalances, such as those involving sodium (Na), develop gradually and usually are not life-threatening

C. Other electrolyte imbalances, such as those involving potassium (K), can quickly become life-threatening if not recognized and treated promptly

D. Changes in serum concentrations of chloride (Cl) alone rarely cause problems; Cl can be depleted by diuretics, especially furosemide; imbalances usually are reflected as metabolic acid-base imbalances; see Chapter 7, sections IV and V

II. Sodium deficit: hyponatremia

A. General information

1. Hyponatremia begins with an excessive Na loss or an excessive water gain in the extracellular fluid (ECF)
2. As ECF osmolality decreases from Na deficiency or water excess, Na moves out of the intracellular fluid (ICF) into the ECF, and water moves into the ICF, which alters ICF osmolality
3. Water movement into the ICF causes cellular swelling and eventually central nervous system (CNS) changes
4. Hyponatremia may result from increased Na and water levels in the ECF with a relatively greater water increase, as in congestive heart failure, liver failure, and nephrotic syndrome
5. Hyponatremia may result from decreased Na and water levels in the ECF with a relatively greater Na decrease

B. Etiology

1. Prolonged diuretic therapy
2. Excessive diaphoresis
3. Insufficient Na intake
4. Excessive Na loss from trauma, such as massive burns
5. Severe gastrointestinal (GI) fluid losses from gastric suctioning or lavage, prolonged vomiting or diarrhea, or laxative abuse
6. Administration of hypotonic fluids
7. Compulsive water drinking linked to a psychological disturbance
8. Labor induction with oxytocin
9. Adrenal insufficiency
10. Na-losing renal disease
11. Cystic fibrosis
12. Alcoholism
13. Syndrome of inappropriate antidiuretic hormone (ADH) secretion (SIADH)
14. Repeated tap water enemas

C. Clinical manifestations
1. Headache
2. Faintness
3. Confusion
4. Muscle cramps
5. Muscle twitching
6. Normal or increased weight
7. Convulsions
8. Coma
9. Irritability
10. Anxiety
11. Hypotension
12. Tachycardia
13. Decreased urine output
14. Decreased tissue turgor

D. Diagnostic findings
1. Serum Na level less than 135 mEq/liter; serum Cl less than 100 mEq/liter
2. Urine specific gravity less than 1.010 (greater than 1.012 in SIADH)
3. Serum osmolality less than 285 mOsm/kg

E. Nursing implications
1. Monitor and record fluid intake and output; relatively greater increases in water in relation to Na will decrease output in relation to intake
2. Restrict fluid intake as ordered; this treatment is the primary one for hyponatremia
3. Administer parenteral fluids as ordered; Na should be administered sparingly to prevent increases in total fluid volume
4. Monitor and record vital signs, particularly blood pressure and pulse rate
5. Assess skin integrity at least every 8 hours
6. Administer intravenous (I.V.) isotonic or hypertonic saline solutions cautiously to avoid inducing hypernatremia from excessive or too-rapid infusion; use an infusion pump
7. Monitor serum Na levels to determine treatment effectiveness
8. Teach the patient and family to use diuretics carefully to avoid excessive Na loss
9. Monitor daily weight for increases linked to water excess
10. Teach the patient and family to follow any Na-restricted diet carefully to ensure low, but still adequate, Na intake

III. Sodium excess: hypernatremia

A. General information
1. Increased serum Na levels usually indicate a water deficit in the ECF, which moves water out of the ICF to equilibrate; increased salt intake also can increase the sodium levels
2. Cellular shrinkage results from increased Na levels in the ECF, increasing serum osmolality, and water movement from the ICF into the ECF
3. Cellular shrinkage in the CNS causes impaired neurologic and cognitive function
4. Hypernatremia usually results in ICF volume deficit

B. Etiology
1. Significantly deficient water intake
2. Hypertonic parenteral fluid administration
3. Hypertonic tube feedings
4. Excessive salt ingestion
5. Severe watery diarrhea or severe insensible water losses, such as from heat stroke or prolonged high fever
6. Major burns
7. Use of inadequately diluted baby formulas
8. Use of high-protein liquid diets without adequate fluid intake
9. Osmotic diuresis, such as in hyperosmolar nonketotic syndrome (HNKS)
10. Diabetes insipidus
11. Aldosteronism

C. Clinical manifestations
1. Extreme thirst
2. Tachycardia
3. Low-grade fever
4. Dry, sticky tongue and oral mucosa
5. Disorientation
6. Hallucinations
7. Lethargy progressing to coma
8. Hyperactive deep tendon reflexes
9. Seizures
10. Coma
11. Hypertension
12. Oliguria or anuria
13. Agitation

D. Diagnostic findings
1. Serum Na level greater than 145 mEq/liter; Cl level elevated
2. Urine specific gravity greater than 1.015
3. Serum osmolality greater than 295 mOsm/kg

E. Nursing implications
1. Monitor and record fluid intake and output; the patient may have seriously decreased output
2. Monitor daily weight for changes
3. Assess for changes in mental function and level of consciousness
4. Monitor and record vital signs, particularly blood pressure, pulse rate, and temperature
5. Cautiously administer ordered parenteral fluids (usually hypotonic Na solution or any hypotonic solution except dextrose 5% in water) to prevent fluid overload and resultant cerebral edema
6. Assess skin and mucous membranes for signs of breakdown and infection
7. Provide thorough oral hygiene to keep mucous membranes moist and to decrease odor
8. Monitor laboratory test results for trends pointing to hypernatremia
9. When a patient is receiving hypertonic fluids, ensure adequate water administration to prevent solute overload; for example, dilute tube feedings and infuse total parenteral nutrition (TPN) at the prescribed rate
10. Teach the patient and family about foods and over-the-counter medications high in Na to prevent accidental overingestion of Na
11. Encourage the patient and family to minimize use of Na in cooking and at the table
12. If necessary, instruct the patient and family about Na-restricted diets to promote compliance

IV. Potassium deficit: hypokalemia

A. General information
1. Hypokalemia usually results from excessive excretion or inadequate intake of K
2. K functions as the major intracellular cation and balances Na in the ECF to maintain the electroneutrality of body fluids
3. K is freely excreted by the kidneys and is not stored by the body
4. About 40 mEq of K are excreted in 1 liter of urine
5. K is also exchanged for the hydrogen (H) ion when changes in the body's acid-base balance indicate a need for cation exchange; K moves into the cells in exchange for H
6. Increased cellular uptake of K occurs in insulin excess, alkalosis, and certain disorders such as renal failure

B. Etiology
1. Prolonged diuretic therapy (for example, with thiazides or furosemide)
2. Inadequate dietary K intake
3. Administration of K-deficient parenteral fluids
4. Severe diaphoresis

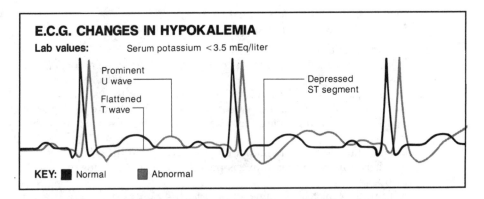

E.C.G. CHANGES IN HYPOKALEMIA

Lab values: Serum potassium <3.5 mEq/liter

Prominent U wave

Flattened T wave

Depressed ST segment

KEY: ■ Normal   ■ Abnormal

5. Severe GI fluid losses from gastric suctioning or lavage, prolonged vomiting or diarrhea, or laxative abuse without K replacement
6. Excessive secretion of endogenous insulin or administration of exogenous insulin
7. Excessive stress (corticosteroid release results in Na retention and K excretion)
8. Alkalosis
9. Hepatic disease
10. Hyperaldosteronism
11. Renal tubular defect (tubular acidosis)
12. Acute alcoholism
13. Cushing syndrome or tumors of the adrenal cortex

C. Clinical manifestations
1. Anorexia
2. Nausea and vomiting
3. Drowsiness and lethargy
4. Leg cramps
5. Muscle weakness, especially in the legs
6. Hyporeflexia
7. Paresthesia
8. Decreased bowel motility (ileus)
9. Hypotension
10. Cardiac ARRHYTHMIAS, such as premature atrial contractions or premature ventricular contractions
11. Coma

D. Diagnostic findings
1. Electrocardiogram (ECG) changes; depressed ST segment, flattened T waves, and U waves present or superimposed on the T waves (see *ECG Changes in Hypokalemia*)
2. Serum K level less than 3.5 mEq/liter
3. Elevated pH and bicarbonate level

4. Urine specific gravity less than 1.010
5. Slightly elevated serum glucose level

E. Nursing implications
   1. Monitor for signs and symptoms of hypokalemia in patients who are at risk
   2. Observe patients receiving diuretics closely because they are more susceptible to hypokalemia; patients receiving digitalis are in danger if hypokalemia occurs because hypokalemia and digitalis cause digitalis toxicity
   3. Monitor fluid intake and output closely; because 40 mEq of K is lost per liter of urine output, diuresis puts the patient at risk for serious K loss
   4. Administer oral K replacements in at least 4 ounces of fluid or with food to prevent gastric irritation
   5. Administer I.V. K supplement infusions cautiously; always dilute and mix thoroughly in adequate amounts of fluid
      a. The usual dose is 20 to 40 mmole/1,000 ml normal saline infused over 1 hour
      b. Such patients should be placed on a cardiac monitor
   6. Never administer K through I.V. push or as a bolus, which could prove fatal
   7. Assess the I.V. infusion site for signs and symptoms of infiltration or pain; high-concentration solutions may cause discomfort and irritation
   8. Monitor heart rate, rhythm, and ECG tracings in a severely hypokalemic patient with a serum K level less than 3 mEq/liter, in a patient receiving greater than 5 mEq of K per hour I.V., and in a patient receiving I.V. K at a concentration greater than 40 mEq K to 1 liter of fluid
   9. Monitor vital signs, particularly pulse rate and blood pressure; postural hypotension may occur with hypokalemia
   10. Monitor serum K levels carefully; keep in mind that relatively minor changes in serum K levels can cause serious cardiac complications
   11. Monitor for signs of metabolic alkalosis, such as irritability and confusion, which may be linked to hypokalemia
   12. Teach the patient and family measures to increase dietary intake of K, especially if the patient is taking a diuretic
   13. Instruct the patient and family in how to properly use oral K supplements

V. Potassium excess: hyperkalemia

A. General information
   1. Hyperkalemia results from impaired renal excretion of K or excessive K intake
   2. Hyperkalemia can also occur in metabolic acidosis; K moves into serum as H moves into cells, lowering the pH

3. Acidosis-associated hyperkalemia involves a movement of K from cells into serum, rather than an increase in total body K levels
4. Excessive serum K levels act as a myocardial depressant, causing decreased heart rate, decreased cardiac output, and possible cardiac arrest
5. Hyperkalemia causes skeletal muscle weakness, usually the initial symptom that causes patients to seek health care assistance
6. Hyperkalemia also causes smooth muscle hyperactivity, particularly in the GI tract, which can result in colic and diarrhea

B. Etiology
 1. Increased dietary K intake, especially with decreased urine output
 2. Excessive administration of K supplements
 3. Excessive use of salt substitutes, most of which use some form of K as a substitute for Na
 4. Use of K-sparing diuretics, such as spironolactone
 5. Severe, widespread cell damage, such as from burns, trauma, crush injuries, intravascular hemolysis, or increased catabolism
 6. Administration of large volumes of blood that is nearing the expiration date ("old" blood undergoes increased cell hemolysis, resulting in the release of K as cells die)
 7. Lysis of tumor cells from chemotherapy (K is released from dying cells into the ECF)
 8. Hyponatremia
 9. Hypoaldosteronism
 10. Metabolic or respiratory acidosis
 11. Acute or chronic renal failure

C. Clinical manifestations
 1. Apathy
 2. Confusion
 3. Paresthesia and numbness in extremities
 4. Abdominal cramps
 5. Nausea
 6. Flaccid muscle paralysis
 7. Diarrhea
 8. Oliguria
 9. Bradycardia
 10. Idioventricular cardiac arrhythmias
 11. Cardiac arrest

D. Diagnostic findings
 1. Serum K level greater than 5.5 mEq/liter
 2. Decreased arterial pH

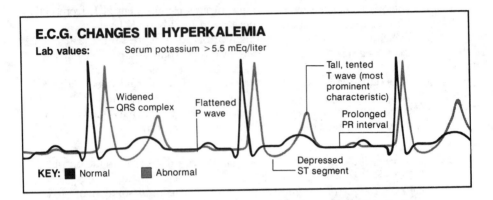

E.C.G. CHANGES IN HYPERKALEMIA

Lab values: Serum potassium > 5.5 mEq/liter

Widened QRS complex

Flattened P wave

Tall, tented T wave (most prominent characteristic)

Prolonged PR interval

Depressed ST segment

KEY: ■ Normal   ■ Abnormal

3. ECG abnormalities; tall, tented T waves; widened QRS complex; prolonged P-R interval; depressed ST segment; and flattened or absent P wave (if not reversed, can lead to asystole) (see *ECG Changes in Hyperkalemia*)

E. Nursing implications
  1. Monitor patients at risk for hyperkalemia, specifically those in acidosis and those receiving K or K-sparing diuretics
  2. Before administering I.V. K supplements, determine whether the patient has a urine output greater than 30 ml/hour; inability to adequately excrete K may lead to dangerously high K levels
  3. Remember that cardiac monitoring and a 12-lead ECG are indicated with elevated serum K levels; a patient with ECG changes may need aggressive treatment to prevent cardiac arrest; the term "symptomatic" hyperkalemia refers to ECG changes that are present with a serum K level greater than 5.5 mEq/liter
  4. Assess cardiovascular status by monitoring pulse rate and rhythm and blood pressure; blood pressure may be elevated initially but may drop as cardiac changes occur, and pulse rate may be slow and regular or irregular, or fast and irregular
  5. Assess for hyperactive bowel sounds and diarrhea
  6. Monitor serum K levels to determine treatment effectiveness
  7. Assess motor and sensory function, especially of the extremities, for changes that may indicate changes in serum K levels
  8. Monitor neurologic status for changes; loss of consciousness may not occur with severe hyperkalemia until cardiac arrest occurs
  9. Be prepared to give calcium gluconate by slow I.V. infusion in acute cases to counteract the myocardial depressant effects of hyperkalemia; the patient must be on a cardiac monitor during administration
  10. Keep in mind that symptomatic acute hyperkalemia may be treated temporarily on an emergency basis by administering dextrose 50% and regular insulin I.V. to facilitate K movement back into the cells

11. Prepare the patient for the possibility of dialysis, either peritoneal or hemodialysis, which may be ordered in acute cases (in acute symptomatic hyperkalemia, only hemodialysis is used)
12. As ordered, administer sodium polystyrene sulfonate (Kayexalate) – a cation-exchange resin – orally or rectally to decrease serum K levels as the K moves into the bowel space and the Na moves into the bowel cell
13. Administer oral sodium polystyrene sulfonate with sorbitol or another osmotic substance to enhance its K-removing action
14. Be aware that oral sodium polystyrene sulfonate should be excreted within 24 hours to prevent bowel perforation; administer soapsuds enemas as necessary to promote excretion
15. Administer rectal sodium polystyrene sulfonate as a retention enema; patients commonly experience cramps or diarrhea, making enema administration and retention difficult; use of an indwelling urinary drainage catheter with the balloon inflated helps with enema administration and retention
16. Monitor for signs of hypernatremia and congestive heart failure in a patient receiving sodium polystyrene sulfonate
17. Administer sodium bicarbonate as ordered to a patient with acidosis to decrease serum K levels by creating alkalosis
18. Teach patients, particularly those with renal failure or renal insufficiency, about foods and fluids high in K and the importance of avoiding them to prevent hyperkalemia
19. Remind patients that most salt substitutes are high in K
20. Be aware that hemolysis of blood samples, either from too tight a tourniquet or too rapid pulling of blood into a vial or syringe, may cause falsely elevated K levels (pseudohyperkalemia); a sample should be redrawn if no clinical symptoms exist

VI. Calcium deficit: hypocalcemia

A. General information
1. Hypocalcemia results from abnormalities of parathyroid hormone secretion or from inadequate dietary intake or excessive losses of bound, ionized (unbound), or total body calcium (Ca)
2. Hypocalcemia usually reflects decreased circulating ionized Ca levels
3. Hypocalcemia can cause skeletal and neuromuscular abnormalities
4. Hypocalcemia impairs clotting mechanisms
5. Because Ca helps maintain cellular integrity, hypocalcemia affects cell membrane integrity and permeability
6. Because one-half of ingested Ca is bound to protein, serum protein abnormalities influence serum Ca levels
7. Because one-half of ionized Ca is absorbed in the gut with vitamin D, GI tract or vitamin D abnormalities decrease serum Ca levels

8. Symptoms of hypocalcemia reflect increased neural excitability and spontaneous stimulation of sensory and motor fibers

B. Etiology
   1. Surgically induced or primary hypoparathyroidism
   2. Acute or chronic renal failure
   3. Chronic malabsorption syndrome
   4. Vitamin D deficiency
   5. Inadequate exposure to ultraviolet light
   6. Chronic insufficient dietary intake of Ca
   7. Hyperphosphatemia
   8. Acute pancreatitis
   9. Administration of large amounts of citrated blood
   10. Alkalosis
   11. Hypoalbuminemia
   12. Hypomagnesemia
   13. Antineoplastic drugs, such as mithramycin and cisplatinum

C. Clinical manifestations
   1. Muscle cramps or tremors
   2. Hyperactive deep tendon reflexes
   3. Paresthesia of the fingers, toes, and face
   4. TETANY
   5. Positive TROUSSEAU'S SIGN
   6. Positive CHVOSTEK'S SIGN
   7. Spasm of laryngeal and bronchial muscles
   8. Spasm of abdominal muscles
   9. Confusion
   10. Moodiness and anxiety
   11. Memory loss
   12. Seizures
   13. Arrhythmias

D. Diagnostic findings
   1. ECG; prolonged Q-T interval and ST segment, (see *ECG Changes in Hypocalcemia*)
   2. Serum Ca level less than 8.5 mg/dl (less than 4.5 mEq/liter)
   3. Ionized Ca level less than 50%
   4. Light precipitation on Sulkowitch's urine test
   5. Prolonged prothrombin time and partial thromboplastin time

E. Nursing implications
   1. Carefully assess patients at increased risk for hypocalcemia, especially after parathyroidectomy or massive transfusions; be especially alert for the coexistence of other electrolyte imbalances, such as hypokalemia and hypomagnesemia
   2. Remember that seizure precautions may be indicated based on the extent of musculoskeletal complications

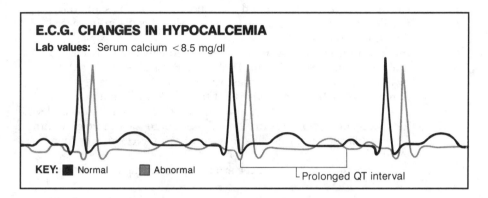

E.C.G. CHANGES IN HYPOCALCEMIA

Lab values: Serum calcium < 8.5 mg/dl

KEY: ■ Normal   ■ Abnormal   └ Prolonged QT interval

3. Institute safety precautions, such as padded bed rails and restraints, to prevent injury, especially if the patient is confused
4. Remember that Ca may be given initially as a slow I.V. bolus, followed by a slow I.V. drip infusion if Ca deficit is acute
5. Administer I.V. Ca replacements carefully, ensuring that the vein is patent; infiltration can cause tissue necrosis and sloughing
6. Place the patient on a cardiac monitor, and observe for changes in heart rate and rhythm
7. Monitor a patient receiving I.V. Ca for arrhythmias, especially if he or she is also taking digitalis (Ca sensitizes the heart to digitalis); too-rapid administration can lead to cardiac arrest; I.V. Ca may be contraindicated in patients receiving digitalis
8. Expect to administer oral Ca supplements or vitamin D for mild to moderate hypocalcemia
9. Assess the patient's nutritional intake for Ca or vitamin D deficiencies; adjust dietary intake to increase Ca
10. Keep calcium gluconate at the bedside of a patient recovering from parathyroid or thyroid surgery to administer if a rapid drop in serum Ca level occurs
11. Teach the patient and family about foods and fluids high in Ca, such as dairy products and green, leafy vegetables
12. Teach the patient and family that exercise enhances Ca mobilization from bone to replenish ECF levels
13. Teach the patient and family that female hormones, such as estrogen, may be administered to maintain adequate Ca levels in patients with osteoporosis

VII. Calcium excess: hypercalcemia

A. General information
   1. Hypercalcemia occurs when the rate of Ca entry into the ECF exceeds the rate of renal Ca excretion

2. Normally, bone resorption and formation occur at the same rate; mobilization of Ca from bone, for any reason, results in increased serum Ca levels
3. Increased intestinal absorption of Ca—from either increased availability, increased vitamin D absorption, or altered GI metabolism—also results in increased serum Ca levels
4. Renal abnormalities (particularly of the tubules) that interfere with secretion and excretion of Ca also can cause increased serum Ca levels
5. Hypercalcemia symptoms are directly related to the degree of serum Ca elevation; severe symptoms may occur with levels greater than 16 mg/dl
6. Patients with metastatic cancer are at especially high risk for hypercalcemia

B. Etiology
1. Excessive intake of Ca supplements
2. Excessive use of Ca-containing antacids (phosphate-binding gels)
3. Prolonged immobility
4. Excessive vitamin D intake
5. Use of thiazide diuretics
6. Primary hyperparathyroidism
7. Metastatic carcinoma
8. Thyrotoxicosis
9. Hypophosphatemia
10. Renal tubular acidosis
11. Milk-alkali syndrome

C. Clinical manifestations
1. Muscle weakness or flaccidity
2. Personality changes, such as neurotic behavior progressing to psychoses
3. Nausea and vomiting
4. Extreme thirst
5. Anorexia
6. Constipation
7. Polyuria
8. Urinary calculi
9. Pathologic fractures and bone cysts
10. Metastatic calcifications, particularly in the cornea and skin (causes itching)
11. Arrhythmias and cardiac arrest
12. Altered level of consciousness, impaired memory, slurred speech
13. Coma

D. Diagnostic findings
1. Serum Ca level greater than 10.5 mg/dl
2. Bone changes on X-ray, such as pathologic fractures

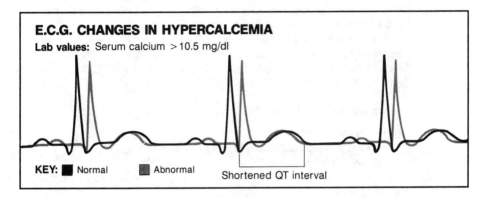

E.C.G. CHANGES IN HYPERCALCEMIA

Lab values: Serum calcium > 10.5 mg/dl

KEY: ■ Normal   ▦ Abnormal   Shortened QT interval

3. Dense precipitation on Sulkowitch's urine test
4. ECG changes; shortened Q-T interval (see *ECG Changes in Hypercalcemia*)

E. Nursing implications
1. Monitor patients at risk for hypercalcemia, especially those with hyperparathyroidism or cancer and those on long-term bed rest
2. Ambulate the patient as soon as possible to prevent Ca mobilization from the bone
3. Have the patient drink 3 to 4 liters of fluids daily (if not contraindicated) to stimulate renal Ca excretion
4. Offer the patient foods or fluids high in Na (if not contraindicated) because the kidneys excrete Ca in favor of Na
5. In a patient with acute moderate to severe hypercalcemia (levels greater than 13 mg/dl), administer I.V. isotonic normal saline solution, usually at a rate of 200 to 500 ml/hour, to reverse dehydration and promote urinary Ca excretion
6. Administer loop diuretics, such as furosemide, to prevent volume overload with I.V. normal saline solution and to increase urinary Ca excretion
7. Remember that calcitonin may be given to lower serum Ca levels temporarily in acute cases if I.V. normal saline solution is ineffective
8. Place the patient on a cardiac monitor to detect arrhythmias
9. In patients with hypercalcemia and low serum phosphorus (P) levels, administer inorganic P salts orally, rectally, or I.V. to lower serum Ca levels by inhibiting bone resorption, reducing Ca absorption, and forming a Ca-P complex
10. Keep in mind that corticosteroids may be used to decrease GI absorption of Ca
11. Monitor serum Ca, P, and Na levels to determine treatment effectiveness and to detect new imbalances resulting from therapy

12. Institute safety precautions, such as restraints and elevated side rails, for a confused and disoriented patient
13. Teach the patient and family signs and symptoms to assess, such as personality changes, muscle weakness, and pathologic fractures
14. Teach the patient to avoid Ca-containing foods and fluids, particularly dairy products, to prevent increased serum Ca levels

VIII. Phosphorus deficit: hypophosphatemia

A. General information
  1. Hypophosphatemia commonly results from decreased intestinal absorption of phosphorus (P)
  2. It also may result from renal wasting of P as a method of controlling acid-base balance or during diuresis
  3. Hypophosphatemia may result from P redistribution from the ECF to the ICF, such as may occur from I.V. glucose administration
  4. P in the form of adenosine triphosphate (ATP) helps maintain the integrity of cell membranes and produces energy within cells
  5. P as 2,3-diphosphoglycerate functions in red blood cells to promote oxygen release to cells
  6. Serum P levels are influenced by diet, parathyroid hormone, and renal function

B. Etiology
  1. Inadequate dietary P intake, such as in malnutrition
  2. Severe, prolonged vomiting
  3. Excessive administration of P-binding gels
  4. Thiazide diuretic therapy
  5. Alcoholism and alcohol withdrawal
  6. Administration of carbohydrates or TPN without P to malnourished patients
  7. I.V. glucose or insulin administration (moves P into skeletal muscle, decreasing serum levels)
  8. Malabsorption syndromes
  9. Hyperparathyroidism
  10. Severe metabolic acidosis, such as in diabetic ketoacidosis
  11. Respiratory alkalosis
  12. Thermal burns
  13. Hypokalemia
  14. Hypomagnesemia
  15. Acute gout
  16. Aldosteronism
  17. Pancreatitis
  18. Renal disease
  19. High Ca intake

C. Clinical manifestations
1. Paresthesia
2. Profound muscle weakness
3. Muscle pain and tenderness
4. Anorexia
5. Malaise
6. Rapid, shallow respirations and potential for respiratory depression
7. Altered level of consciousness
8. Seizures
9. Nystagmus and unequal pupils
10. Heart failure
11. Hemolytic anemia
12. Platelet dysfunction
13. Skeletal abnormalities

D. Diagnostic findings
1. Serum P level less than 3 mg/dl
2. Hypercalciuria
3. Elevated creatine phosphokinase (CPK) levels when serum P levels are less than 1 mg/dl for 1 day or more

E. Nursing implications
1. Monitor patients at risk for hypophosphatemia, especially those receiving TPN without P replacement
2. Assess for paresthesia, particularly in the circumoral area—an early sign of hypophosphatemia
3. Initiate safety precautions for a patient with confusion or decreased level of consciousness
4. Assess for signs and symptoms of infection; in hypophosphatemia, granulocytes have less ability to fight foreign bodies
5. Assess a patient with hypophosphatemia for signs and symptoms of hypercalcemia, such as urinary calculi, because of the reciprocal relationship between Ca and P
6. Expect to administer oral P supplements to a patient with mild to moderate hypophosphatemia
7. Use caution when administering parenteral P to a patient with severe hypophosphatemia; hypocalcemia may occur as P levels rise
8. Remember that malnourished patients should be re-fed gradually to avoid hypophosphatemia resulting from I.V. glucose administration
9. Instruct the patient and family in measures to increase dietary P intake

IX. Phosphorus excess: hyperphosphatemia

A. General information
1. Hyperphosphatemia most commonly results from decreased P excretion in renal disease

2. Of the remaining cases of hyperphosphatemia, about one-half have no explainable etiology; some cases may be attributed to increased dietary P intake

3. Lysis of tumor cells during cancer chemotherapy can result in P redistribution from the ICF to the ECF, possibly causing hyperphosphatemia

4. Laxatives and P-based enemas may increase P absorption from the GI tract

B. Etiology
   1. Acute or chronic renal failure
   2. Excessive dietary P intake
   3. Excessive vitamin D use
   4. Hypoparathyroidism
   5. Cancer chemotherapy
   6. Excessive use of laxatives and P-based enemas

C. Clinical manifestations
   1. Tetany
   2. Circumoral paresthesia
   3. Muscle spasms
   4. Seizures (chronic P increase may decrease Ca levels)
   5. Soft tissue calcification (with long-standing hyperphosphatemia)

D. Diagnostic findings
   1. Serum P level greater than 4.5 mg/dl
   2. Decreased serum Ca level

E. Nursing implications
   1. Monitor patients at risk, particularly those with hypocalcemia
   2. Initiate seizure precautions in patients with elevated P levels
   3. Monitor for neuromuscular irritability, which accompanies high P levels
   4. Remember that P-binding antacids, such as aluminum hydroxide gel, may be administered to lower serum P levels
   5. Keep in mind that acetazolamide may be administered to increase urinary P excretion; dialysis can also be used for hyperphosphatemia
   6. Administer Ca supplements to promote elevation of serum Ca levels, which lowers serum P levels
   7. Teach the patient and family to avoid foods and fluids high in P, such as cheeses, nuts, whole-grain cereals, dried fruits, and vegetables
   8. Teach the patient and family to avoid excessive use of enemas and laxatives containing P

X. Magnesium deficit: hypomagnesemia

A. General information

1. Hypomagnesemia results from excessive magnesium (Mg) loss from increased renal excretion or GI fluid losses, insufficient dietary Mg intake, or movement of Mg from the ECF to the ICF

2. Mg, the second most abundant intracellular cation, is essential for neuromuscular integration; hypomagnesemia increases muscle cell irritability and contractility

3. Mg also activates enzyme systems and contributes to intracellular biochemical reactions

4. Hypomagnesemia causes decreased blood pressure and may result in ventricular arrhythmias

5. Hypomagnesemia and hypokalemia, which often occur simultaneously, produce similar signs and symptoms

B. Etiology

1. Excessive dietary intake of Ca or vitamin D

2. Severe GI fluid losses from gastric suctioning or lavage, prolonged vomiting or diarrhea, or laxative abuse

3. Prolonged, excessive diuretic therapy

4. Administration of I.V. fluids or TPN without Mg replacement

5. Prolonged malnutrition or starvation

6. Malabsorption syndromes

7. Ulcerative colitis

8. Hypercalcemia

9. Hypoparathyroidism

10. Hypoaldosteronism

11. High-dose steroid use

12. Cancer chemotherapy

13. Gentamicin therapy

14. Burns and debridement therapy

15. Sepsis

16. Pancreatitis

17. Diabetic ketoacidosis

18. Chronic alcoholism and alcohol withdrawal

19. Pregnancy-induced hypertension

C. Clinical manifestations

1. Tachycardia and other arrhythmias and hypotension

2. Tremors

3. Tetany

4. Hyperactive deep tendon reflexes

5. Positive Chvostek's and Trousseau's signs

6. Memory loss

7. Emotional lability

8. Confusion

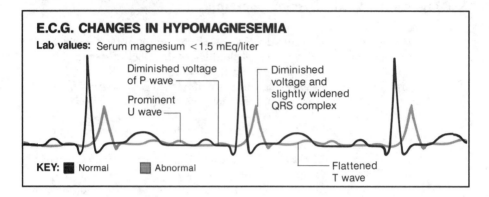

E.C.G. CHANGES IN HYPOMAGNESEMIA

Lab values: Serum magnesium < 1.5 mEq/liter

Diminished voltage of P wave

Prominent U wave

Diminished voltage and slightly widened QRS complex

Flattened T wave

KEY: ■ Normal ▨ Abnormal

9. Dizziness
10. Anorexia
11. Nausea
12. Hallucinations
13. Seizures
14. Coma

D. Diagnostic findings
   1. Serum Mg level less than 1.5 mEq/liter (clinical manifestations occur at about 1 mEq/liter)
   2. Hypocalcemia
   3. Hypokalemia
   4. ECG changes; flattened T wave, slightly widened QRS complex, diminished voltage of P waves and QRS complex, and prominent U wave (see *ECG Changes in Hypomagnesemia*)

E. Nursing implications
   1. Monitor patients at risk for hypomagnesemia, particularly those with hypokalemia and those receiving TPN without Mg replacement
   2. Monitor a patient taking digitalis for signs of digitalis toxicity; the risk of digitalis toxicity is increased in hypomagnesemia resulting from the body's retention of digitalis
   3. Institute cardiac monitoring in a patient with severe hypomagnesemia
   4. Initiate seizure precautions to prevent patient injury
   5. Monitor for signs and symptoms of hypomagnesemia during prolonged infusion of Mg-free I.V. fluids
   6. Remember that hypomagnesemia may be treated with oral, intramuscular, or I.V. Mg salts
   7. Monitor serum Ca levels during Mg replacement therapy because hypocalcemia can occur at this time
   8. Administer I.V. Mg slowly because too-rapid infusion can cause cardiac or respiratory arrest

9. During I.V. Mg therapy, monitor urine output; it should be at least 100 ml every 4 hours for adequate renal Mg elimination
10. Assess deep tendon reflexes during long-term I.V. Mg therapy; if reflexes are absent, hold the dose and notify the doctor
11. For a patient experiencing seizures, administer a 10% Mg solution at a rate no greater than 1.5 ml/minute
12. Monitor serum Mg and K levels to evaluate treatment effectiveness
13. Assess for laryngeal stridor, which may indicate the onset of airway obstruction with hypomagnesemia
14. Initiate safety precautions, such as elevated bed rails and restraints, for a confused patient
15. Monitor for dysphagia, especially when giving medications or foods, because swallowing may be impaired
16. When hypomagnesemia is suspected as the cause of an arrhythmia, also assess the patient for signs of hypokalemia
17. Teach the patient and family about the dangers of diuretic abuse and its link to hypomagnesemia
18. Teach the patient and family about foods high in Mg, such as green vegetables, nuts, beans, and fruits

XI. Magnesium excess: hypermagnesemia

A. General information
1. Hypermagnesemia usually results from renal failure
2. Excessive Mg intake commonly involves over-the-counter medications or parenteral Mg
3. Mg produces a sedative effect on the neuromuscular junction, inhibits acetylcholine release, and diminishes muscle cell excitability
4. Hypermagnesemia can cause hypotension and possibly cardiac arrest

B. Etiology
1. Renal failure
2. Excessive use of Mg-containing antacids or laxatives
3. Excessive administration of parenteral Mg
4. Untreated diabetic ketoacidosis
5. Hypoadrenalism
6. Hemodialysis using hard water high in Mg

C. Clinical manifestations
1. Lethargy and drowsiness
2. Depressed neuromuscular activity
3. Depressed respirations
4. Sensation of warmth throughout the body
5. Hypoactive deep tendon reflexes
6. Hypotension
7. Bradycardia
8. Cardiac arrest

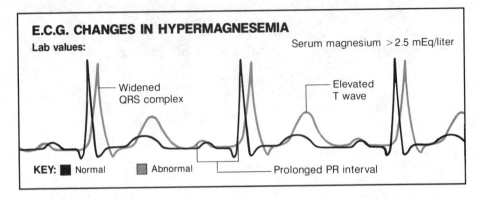

E.C.G. CHANGES IN HYPERMAGNESEMIA
Lab values: Serum magnesium >2.5 mEq/liter

Widened
QRS complex

Elevated
T wave

KEY: ■ Normal   ▨ Abnormal   └─── Prolonged PR interval

    9. Coma

D. Diagnostic findings
    1. Serum Mg level greater than 3 mEq/liter
    2. ECG changes; widened QRS complex, prolonged P-R interval, and
       elevated T wave (see *ECG Changes in Hypermagnesemia*)

E. Nursing implications
    1. Monitor patients at risk, especially those with conditions predisposing
       to hypermagnesemia, such as renal failure
    2. Monitor vital signs—particularly blood pressure, which can drop
       precipitously, and respirations, which may be depressed and can
       progress to apnea
    3. Assess neuromuscular status for deficits; evaluate reflexes, grip
       strength, and respiratory muscle function
    4. In a patient with renal failure, check for any standing orders for Mg-
       containing medication, such as laxatives or antacids; administer them
       cautiously
    5. Institute cardiac monitoring for a patient with serum Mg levels greater
       than 7 mEq/liter because this patient has an increased risk for cardiac
       arrest
    6. Be prepared to administer calcium gluconate, an Mg antagonist, to
       temporarily relieve symptoms in an emergency
    7. Monitor serum Mg levels for changes to evaluate the patient's response
       to therapy
    8. Teach the patient and family to minimize intake of foods high in Mg,
       such as green vegetables, nuts, beans, and fruits

XII. Patients at risk for electrolyte imbalances

A. General information
    1. Patients vary in their susceptibility to electrolyte imbalances

2. Age- and illness-related physiologic changes affect the body's ability to compensate for imbalances
3. Because of the close association between water and electrolytes, patients at risk for water imbalances are also at risk for electrolyte imbalances
4. Three groups of patients at highest risk are infants and children, older adults, and chronically ill patients

B. Infants and children
1. Infants and children are at high risk for elevated electrolyte levels from electrolyte replacement therapy
2. Feeding an infant improperly diluted infant formula can cause renal damage from a hypertonic solute load
3. Feeding an infant cow's milk rather than formula or breast milk can cause hyperphosphatemia because of the higher P level in cow's milk

C. Older adults
1. Older adults taking diuretics or digitalis preparations are at particular risk for electrolyte imbalances, especially hypokalemia
2. Digitalis toxicity is a particular problem in this age group because K, Ca, and Mg imbalances predispose to this condition
3. Inadequate water intake predisposes an older adult to excessive solute loads
4. Inadequate nutrition predisposes an older adult to electrolyte deficits, which may be aggravated by diuretic therapy

D. Chronically ill patients
1. Many chronic diseases—particularly renal failure, diabetes mellitus, and endocrine disorders—are considered etiologic factors in various electrolyte imbalances
2. Chronic illness impairs the body's ability to compensate for imbalances; monitor these patients closely

Points to remember

Sodium (Na) imbalances are usually accompanied by fluid imbalances.

Potassium (K) imbalances can lead to life-threatening cardiac dysfunction.

Calcium (Ca) imbalances are associated with neuromuscular problems.

ECG changes occur in K, Ca, and magnesium (Mg) imbalances.

Infants and young children, older adults, and chronically ill patients have an increased risk for electrolyte imbalances.

Glossary

The following terms are defined in Appendix A, page 127.

arrhythmia

Chvostek's sign

tetany

Trousseau's sign

Study questions

To evaluate your understanding of this chapter, answer the following questions in the space provided; then compare your responses with the correct answers in Appendix B, page 132.

1. What are three key causes of hyponatremia? _____

_____

_____

2. What is the primary treatment for hyponatremia? _____

_____

_____

3. What are four clinical manifestations of hypernatremia? _____

_____

_____

4. Approximately how much K is excreted in one liter of urine? _____

_____

_____

5. What ECG changes might the nurse see in a patient with hypokalemia?

_____

_____

6. How is K replacement therapy administered? _____

_____

_____

7. What effect does hyperkalemia have on the heart? _____

_____

_____

8. What must the nurse assess if the patient with hypocalcemia is receiving I.V. Ca and also digitalis? _____

_____

Study questions *(continued)*

9. From what does hypophosphatemia commonly result? _____

_____

_____

10. What patient teaching information should the nurse include for the patient with hypomagnesemia? _____

_____

11. What ECG changes are seen in hypermagnesemia? _____

_____

_____

12. Why should an infant not be fed cow's milk? _____

_____

_____

CHAPTER 7

Acid-Base Imbalances

Learning objectives

Check off the following items once you've mastered them:

☐ List the four major types of acid-base imbalances.

☐ Describe the major alteration in carbon dioxide associated with respiratory acidosis and alkalosis.

☐ Describe the major alteration in bicarbonate associated with metabolic acidosis and alkalosis.

☐ State the nursing implications for each acid-base imbalance.

I. Introduction

A. Acid-base imbalances are common clinical conditions that accompany any disorder

B. The hydrogen (H) cation influences both electrolyte balance and acid-base balance

C. H ion concentration (pH) is measured through arterial blood gas (ABG) analysis

D. Acid-base imbalances are categorized into four major types: respiratory acidosis, respiratory alkalosis, metabolic acidosis, and metabolic alkalosis

E. These major imbalances can occur in three forms: primary, combined or mixed, and compensated

F. *Primary imbalances* originate from an acute condition, such as respiratory acidosis resulting from HYPERVENTILATION syndrome

G. *Combined or mixed imbalances* involve both a metabolic and a respiratory imbalance occurring at the same time; combined or mixed imbalances occur when:
   1. One disturbance results in acidosis; the other results in alkalosis
   2. Both disturbances are acidosis
   3. Both disturbances are alkalosis

H. *Compensated imbalances* involve the body's attempt to bring the pH back to normal after a primary imbalance has occurred; the body compensates for a primary imbalance by initiating the opposite imbalance; compensated imbalances usually are associated with chronic disorders, such as chronic obstructive pulmonary disease (COPD)

I. The body responds to an acid-base imbalance with a physiologic process known as *compensation*
   1. Respiratory imbalances are compensated for by the renal system
   2. Metabolic imbalances are compensated for by the respiratory system

II. Respiratory acidosis

A. General information
   1. Respiratory acidosis is a primary acid-base imbalance resulting from altered alveolar ventilation leading to carbon dioxide (CO_2) retention (see *Respiratory Acidosis: ABG Findings*)
   2. Alveolar HYPOVENTILATION is the most common cause of respiratory acidosis
   3. Abnormally slow or shallow respirations or poor alveolar ventilation resulting in inadequate gas exchange causes CO_2 to accumulate in the lungs and the serum, increasing the levels of carbonic acid (H_2CO_3) circulating in the blood and lowering pH

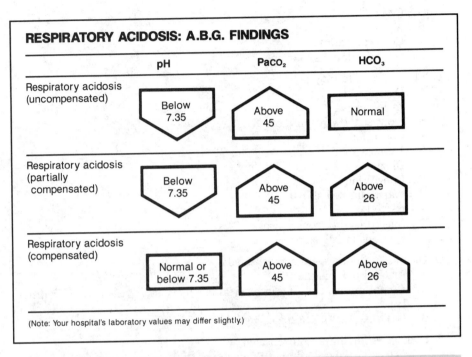

RESPIRATORY ACIDOSIS: A.B.G. FINDINGS

	pH	Paco₂	HCO₃
Respiratory acidosis (uncompensated)	Below 7.35	Above 45	Normal
Respiratory acidosis (partially compensated)	Below 7.35	Above 45	Above 26
Respiratory acidosis (compensated)	Normal or below 7.35	Above 45	Above 26

(Note: Your hospital's laboratory values may differ slightly.)

    4. Low arterial pH and elevated serum CO_2 levels (hypercapnia) constitute respiratory acidosis
    5. Respiratory acidosis may be acute, as in sudden ventilatory failure, or chronic, as in emphysema
    6. The body attempts to compensate for respiratory acidosis by increasing the renal reabsorption of bicarbonate (HCO_3)

B. Etiology
    1. Alveolar hypoventilation
    2. Acute abdominal distention (inhibits pulmonary excursion)
    3. Respiratory arrest
    4. Overdose of sedatives or anesthetic
    5. Airway obstruction
    6. COPD
    7. Congestive heart failure
    8. Pneumonia
    9. Cardiac arrest
    10. Pneumothorax or hydrothorax
    11. Chest wall injury, such as fractured ribs
    12. Amyotrophic lateral sclerosis
    13. Pulmonary fibrosis
    14. Pickwickian syndrome

15. Cystic fibrosis
16. Myasthenia gravis
17. Cerebral trauma
18. Guillain-Barré syndrome

C. Clinical manifestations
1. Dyspnea
2. Tachycardia
3. Slow, shallow respirations
4. Confusion
5. Tremors
6. Dizziness
7. Convulsions
8. Warm, flushed skin
9. ASTERIXIS
10. Altered level of consciousness
11. Cyanosis (a late sign)

D. Diagnostic findings — uncompensated
1. Arterial pH less than 7.35
2. Partial pressure of CO_2 in arterial blood ($PaCO_2$) greater than 45 mm Hg
3. HCO_3 level 22 to 26 mEq/liter

E. Diagnostic findings — compensated
1. Arterial pH borderline (7.35 or lower)
2. $PaCO_2$ greater than 45 mm Hg
3. HCO_3 level greater than 26 mEq/liter

F. Nursing implications
1. Encourage the patient to turn, cough, and breathe deeply every 2 hours, which improves ventilation; chest physiotherapy may also be ordered
2. Maintain a patent airway through the use of measures such as suctioning to prevent CO_2 retention
3. Monitor ABG levels for changes in pH and CO_2
4. Monitor vital signs, particularly respiratory rate and depth, for changes that may indicate worsening acidosis
5. Position the patient in the semi-Fowler's or orthopneic position to ease breathing
6. Ensure that the patient drinks 2 to 3 liters of fluids per day (unless contraindicated) to help liquefy secretions, aid their expulsion, and promote adequate CO_2 exchange
7. Administer supplemental oxygen as ordered; do so cautiously in a patient with COPD because excessive oxygen decreases or completely depresses the ventilatory drive and may worsen acidosis
8. Monitor serum potassium (K) levels for hyperkalemia because K moves out of the cell during respiratory acidosis

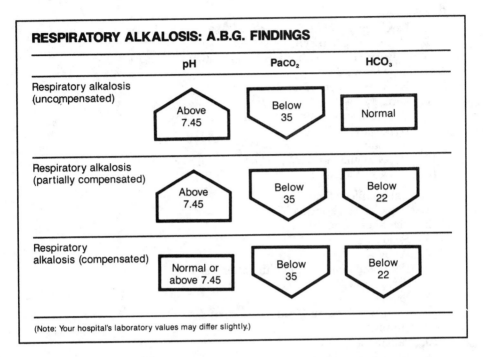

RESPIRATORY ALKALOSIS: A.B.G. FINDINGS

	pH	Paco₂	HCO₃
Respiratory alkalosis (uncompensated)	Above 7.45	Below 35	Normal
Respiratory alkalosis (partially compensated)	Above 7.45	Below 35	Below 22
Respiratory alkalosis (compensated)	Normal or above 7.45	Below 35	Below 22

(Note: Your hospital's laboratory values may differ slightly.)

9. Administer medications, as ordered, to treat the underlying respiratory dysfunction—for example, bronchodilators for bronchospasms and antibiotics for respiratory infection
10. Administer sedatives cautiously; many sedatives depress the respiratory drive, which can lead to CO_2 accumulation
11. Provide emotional support and reassurance to the patient, who likely will be quite anxious
12. Assist with intubation if the patient remains unable to ventilate adequately

III. Respiratory alkalosis

A. General information
1. Respiratory alkalosis occurs when alveolar hyperventilation results in decreased serum CO_2 levels (hypocapnia), causing excessive CO_2 exhalation (see *Respiratory Alkalosis: ABG Findings*)
2. Decreased serum CO_2 levels lead to decreased H_2CO_3 production and, in turn, increased arterial pH
3. Hyperventilation is the most common cause of respiratory alkalosis
4. The body attempts to compensate for respiratory alkalosis by increasing renal excretion of HCO_3 (can take 24 to 48 hours)

B. Etiology
1. Psychogenic conditions, such as hysteria or acute anxiety
2. Hyperventilation syndrome
3. Overventilation with mechanical ventilator
4. Aspirin overdose
5. Fever from septicemia
6. Severe pain
7. Central nervous system trauma or lesions
8. Hypoxia
9. Pregnancy
10. Hyperventilation during labor and delivery
11. THYROTOXICOSIS

C. Clinical manifestations
1. Rapid, deep respirations
2. Light-headedness
3. Headache
4. Vertigo
5. Decreased concentration and attention span
6. Paresthesia
7. Tetany
8. Carpopedal spasm (Trousseau's sign)
9. Tinnitus
10. Palpitations
11. Dry mouth
12. Blurred vision
13. Syncope
14. Convulsions and coma
15. Hyperactive deep tendon reflexes
16. Twitching

D. Diagnostic findings – uncompensated
1. $PaCO_2$ level less than 35 mm Hg
2. Arterial pH greater than 7.45
3. Partial pressure of oxygen in arterial blood (PaO_2) normal or elevated (80 to 100)
4. HCO_3 level 22 to 26 mEq/liter

E. Diagnostic findings – compensated
1. $PaCO_2$ level less than 35 mm Hg
2. Arterial pH borderline (7.45 or slightly higher)
3. HCO_3 level less than 22 mEq/liter
4. Serum K level below 3.8 mEq/liter
5. Urine pH alkaline (above 8)
6. Serum calcium (Ca) level below 7 mg/dl

F. Nursing implications
1. Monitor vital signs, specifically respiratory rate and depth

2. Instruct the patient to breathe slowly and less deeply to decrease CO_2 loss
3. As necessary, have the patient breathe into a paper bag or use a rebreather mask to rebreathe CO_2
4. Administer sedatives, as ordered, to slow the respiratory rate; monitor the patient carefully to guard against respiratory depression and CO_2 retention
5. Intervene as necessary to correct the underlying cause of hyperventilation, such as pain or anxiety
6. Monitor ABG values, particularly $PaCO_2$ levels, to evaluate the effectiveness of interventions
7. If the patient is intubated, adjust mechanical ventilator settings to decrease ventilatory rate and depth
8. Monitor serum K levels, especially in a patient with chronic hyperventilation, because K is exchanged for H ions and moves from the extracellular to the intracellular space, resulting in low serum levels
9. Monitor laboratory results for values indicating compensation, such as decreased HCO_3 levels and normalization of pH; such values will not appear until at least 24 hours after onset of hyperventilation
10. Provide emotional support and reassurance to help decrease anxiety

IV. Metabolic acidosis

A. General information
   1. Metabolic acidosis results from excessive accumulation of fixed acids or loss of fixed bases in body fluids (see *Metabolic Acidosis: ABG Findings*, page 80)
   2. Fixed acids, such as hydrochloric acid (HCl), are produced by metabolism or ingested foods
   3. Chloride (Cl), a component of HCl, competes with HCO_3 for combination with sodium (Na); excessive Cl retention or ingestion increases fixed acid production; the kidneys' inability to retain sufficient HCO_3 to compensate results in an excess of H ions and, eventually, metabolic acidosis
   4. The major sign of metabolic acidosis is decreased arterial pH accompanied by decreased arterial HCO_3 levels
   5. Metabolic acidosis never results from a respiratory problem—with the exception of lactic acidosis from anaerobic metabolism (lack of available oxygen at the cellular level)
   6. Increased levels of circulating H ions result in rapid stimulation of peripheral chemoreceptors, which increases the respiratory rate within minutes of the onset of acidosis

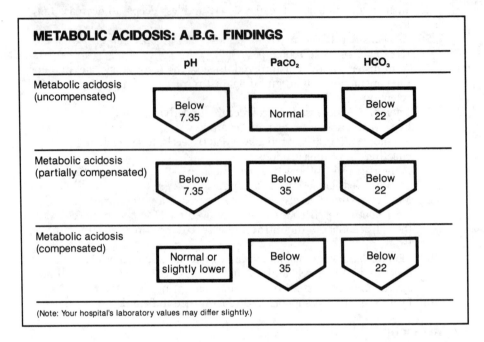

METABOLIC ACIDOSIS: A.B.G. FINDINGS

	pH	Paco₂	HCO₃
Metabolic acidosis (uncompensated)	Below 7.35	Normal	Below 22
Metabolic acidosis (partially compensated)	Below 7.35	Below 35	Below 22
Metabolic acidosis (compensated)	Normal or slightly lower	Below 35	Below 22

(Note: Your hospital's laboratory values may differ slightly.)

7. The body attempts to compensate for metabolic acidosis through hyperventilation, which results in decreased PaCO₂ levels; respiratory compensation begins within minutes but takes several hours to take full effect

B. Etiology
   1. Diabetic ketoacidosis
   2. Salicylate toxicity
   3. Acute or chronic renal failure
   4. Diuretic therapy resulting in excessive HCO₃ loss through the kidneys
   5. Total parenteral nutrition therapy
   6. Prolonged, severe diarrhea
   7. Fistula drainage, for example, pancreatic
   8. Use of carbonic anhydrase inhibitors such as acetazolamide (Diamox)
   9. Alcohol intoxication
   10. Starvation
   11. Hypoxia
   12. Decreased tissue perfusion, such as from trauma or burns
   13. High-fat diet
   14. Excessive gain of Cl, such as from the administration of ammonium chloride

C. Clinical manifestations
   1. KUSSMAUL RESPIRATIONS

2. Lethargy
3. Drowsiness
4. Confusion
5. Headache
6. Flushed, warm, dry skin
7. Fruity breath
8. Peripheral vasodilation
9. Nausea and vomiting
10. Twitching
11. Convulsions
12. Stupor
13. Coma

D. Diagnostic findings — uncompensated
1. Arterial pH level less than 7.35
2. Arterial HCO_3 level less than 22 mEq/liter
3. $PaCO_2$ level 35 to 45 mm Hg
4. Base excess negative
5. Serum CO_2 level less than 18 mEq/liter

E. Diagnostic findings — compensated
1. Arterial pH borderline (7.35 or slightly lower)
2. Arterial HCO_3 level less than 22 mEq/liter
3. $PaCO_2$ level less than 35 mm Hg
4. Base excess negative
5. Serum K level greater than 5.5 mEq/liter
6. Urine pH less than or equal to 4.5

F. Nursing implications
1. Monitor patients at risk for metabolic acidosis, especially those with diabetes mellitus, sepsis, or shock
2. Monitor vital signs, particularly respiratory rate and depth
3. Monitor ABG values, particularly pH, because small decreases in pH indicate large increases in H ion concentration
4. Monitor HCO_3 and K levels; low HCO_3 and high K levels may be an early indicator of acidosis
5. Administer sodium bicarbonate ($NaHCO_3$) cautiously through an existing I.V. line in a large vein
6. Institute cardiac monitoring for a patient with elevated serum K levels
7. As necessary, intervene to correct the underlying cause of acidosis; in many cases, correction of the underlying problem will resolve acidosis, precluding the need for more aggressive intervention, such as $NaHCO_3$ administration
8. As ordered, administer I.V. fluids containing lactate, unless contraindicated; lactate is converted to HCO_3 in the liver

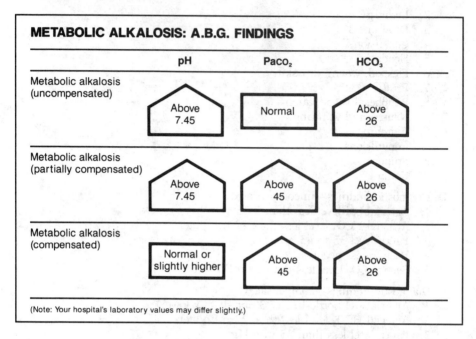

METABOLIC ALKALOSIS: A.B.G. FINDINGS

	pH	Paco₂	HCO₃
Metabolic alkalosis (uncompensated)	Above 7.45	Normal	Above 26
Metabolic alkalosis (partially compensated)	Above 7.45	Above 45	Above 26
Metabolic alkalosis (compensated)	Normal or slightly higher	Above 45	Above 26

(Note: Your hospital's laboratory values may differ slightly.)

9. In a diabetic patient with metabolic acidosis linked to hyperglycemia, administer insulin and normal saline solution to correct hyperglycemia; remember that insulin administration also will lower serum K levels
10. Administer I.V. fluids and oxygen to correct lactic acidosis linked to overexertion by decreasing hypoxemia and triggering a conversion to aerobic metabolism
11. In renal failure, drug overdose, or poisoning, expect to assist with peritoneal dialysis or hemodialysis to correct pH
12. In a patient with chronic acidosis, provide a diet high in carbohydrates and low in fat, which will decrease metabolic waste products and thus ameliorate acidosis

V. Metabolic alkalosis

A. General information
1. Metabolic alkalosis results from excessive accumulation of fixed bases or excessive loss of fixed acids in body fluids (see *Metabolic Alkalosis: ABG Findings*)
2. A major cause of metabolic alkalosis is loss of a fixed acid, such as HCl, from the stomach, either through nasogastric (NG) suctioning or excessive vomiting
3. Loss of a fixed acid increases the pH

4. As pH increases, H ion concentration decreases
5. As H ion concentration decreases, more H_2CO_3 dissociates and HCO_3 concentration increases through renal reabsorption
6. This process results in increased renal excretion of H, Cl, and K
7. Cl competes with HCO_3 for combination with Na; when Cl levels fall, HCO_3 levels rise in compensation to balance Na
8. The body attempts to compensate for metabolic alkalosis through hypoventilation
9. Stimulation of chemoreceptors is decreased, slowing respiratory rate and conserving CO_2

B. Etiology
1. Excessive administration or ingestion of HCO_3
2. Excessive loss of H ions from NG suctioning or vomiting
3. Prolonged diuretic therapy, particularly K-wasting diuretics
4. $NaHCO_3$ administration during cardiopulmonary resuscitation
5. Hypokalemia
6. Cushing's syndrome
7. Hyperaldosteronism

C. Clinical manifestations
1. Decreased respiratory rate and depth
2. Dizziness
3. Paresthesia in fingers and toes
4. CIRCUMORAL PARESTHESIA
5. Carpopedal spasm
6. Muscle hypertonicity
7. Nausea and vomiting
8. Confusion
9. Irritability
10. Agitation
11. Convulsions
12. Coma

D. Diagnostic findings – uncompensated
1. Arterial pH greater than 7.45
2. Arterial HCO_3 level greater than 26 mEq/liter
3. $PaCO_2$ level 35 to 45 mm Hg
4. Base excess positive
5. Serum CO_2 level greater than 28 mEq/liter

E. Diagnostic findings – compensated
1. Arterial pH borderline (7.45 or slightly higher)
2. Arterial HCO_3 levels greater than 26 mEq/liter
3. $PaCO_2$ level greater than 45 mm Hg
4. Base excess positive
5. Serum K and Cl levels (relative to Na) decreased

F. Nursing implications
   1. Monitor patients at risk for metabolic alkalosis, particularly those with gastric fluid losses from long-term NG suctioning or vomiting
   2. Assess fluid intake and output to determine the amount of gastric fluid loss
   3. Monitor vital signs, especially respirations, which will usually decrease as the body attempts to conserve CO_2
   4. As necessary, intervene to correct the underlying cause of the imbalance; for example, control vomiting by administering an antiemetic
   5. Administer I.V. fluid and electrolyte supplements, as ordered, to replace fluid volume, K, and Cl losses; monitor electrolyte studies to prevent overreplacement
   6. Supply sufficient Cl to enable renal absorption of Na with Cl and subsequent renal excretion of excessive HCO_3
   7. Monitor heart rate and rhythm to detect hypokalemia; a 12-lead ECG may be indicated
   8. Warn the patient and family about the dangers of excessive HCO_3 ingestion; explain that alkalosis can develop from overuse of antacids or $NaHCO_3$
   9. Teach a patient taking a K-wasting diuretic to watch for and report symptoms of hypokalemia, such as weakness and excessive urine output; teach the patient and family how to replace K by either increased dietary intake or oral supplements

Points to remember

Respiratory acidosis results from carbon dioxide (CO_2) retention, most commonly from hypoventilation.

Respiratory alkalosis results from excessive CO_2 exhalation, most commonly from hyperventilation.

Metabolic acidosis results from excessive accumulation of fixed acids or excessive loss of fixed bases.

Metabolic alkalosis results from excessive loss of fixed acids or excessive accumulation of fixed bases.

Glossary

The following terms are defined in Appendix A, page 127.

asterixis   hypoventilation

circumoral paresthesia   Kussmaul respirations

hyperventilation   thyrotoxicosis

Study questions

To evaluate your understanding of this chapter, answer the following questions in the space provided; then compare your responses with the correct answers in Appendix B, page 133.

1. What two findings constitute respiratory acidosis? _____

   _____

   _____

2. What is the goal of nursing interventions for a patient with respiratory acidosis? _____

   _____

3. How does the body attempt to compensate for respiratory acidosis?

   _____

   _____

4. When assessing the patient with uncompensated respiratory alkalosis, the nurse would expect to see what ABG findings? _____

   _____

5. What simple intervention can the nurse use to help the patient who is hyperventilating and experiencing respiratory alkalosis? _____

   _____

6. How does the body attempt to compensate for metabolic acidosis?

   _____

   _____

7. How can the nurse intervene for the patient with chronic metabolic acidosis?

   _____

   _____

Study questions (continued)

8. What are four key etiologic reasons for developing metabolic alkalosis?

   _____

   _____

9. What ABG findings would the nurse expect to see for the patient with uncompensated metabolic alkalosis? _____

   _____

10. Which diagnostic findings commonly are seen in metabolic acidosis?

    _____

    _____

CHAPTER 8

Fluid and Electrolyte Replacement Therapy

Learning objectives

Check off the following items once you've mastered them:

☐ List the administration routes for pure water.

☐ List two examples of isotonic and hypotonic crystalloid solutions.

☐ Compare and contrast colloids and blood products.

☐ Discuss the nursing implications associated with each route of fluid and electrolyte replacement therapy.

I. Introduction

A. Fluid and electrolyte replacement therapy is aimed at restoring and maintaining homeostasis

B. Goals of replacement therapy include correcting fluid and electrolyte losses, meeting daily fluid and electrolyte needs, preventing new imbalances, and preserving renal function

C. The type of fluid or electrolyte selected for replacement is determined after the type of fluid or electrolyte imbalance is established

D. Methods of fluid and electrolyte replacement therapy include oral and gastric feedings and parenteral therapy

E. Factors affecting choice of replacement therapy include the patient's overall health status, the patient's renal and cardiovascular status, the patient's age, the patient's usual maintenance requirements, the type of imbalance, and the severity of imbalance

F. Administration routes include the following:
1. Oral route is defined as the oral ingestion of fluids and electrolytes as liquids or solids administered directly into the gastrointestinal (GI) tract
2. Nasogastric (NG) route is defined as instillation of fluids and electrolytes through feeding tubes, such as NG, GASTROSTOMY, and jejunostomy tubes
3. The intravenous (I.V.) route is defined as the administration of fluids and electrolytes directly into the bloodstream; this route may be accomplished by continuous infusion, bolus, or I.V. push injection through a peripheral or central venous site

G. Replacement therapy fluids are categorized by their concentration (tonicity); they are usually prepared in isotonic, hypotonic, and hypertonic concentrations

H. *Isotonic* solutions have the same osmolality as plasma, approximately 285 to 295 mEq/liter
1. Infusion of isotonic fluids does not alter vascular space osmolality
2. Isotonic fluids expand the intracellular and extracellular spaces equally
3. The degree of intracellular fluid (ICF) and extracellular fluid (ECF) expansion correlates with the amount of fluid infused
4. Examples of isotonic solutions include Ringer's solution and lactated Ringer's solution

I. *Hypotonic* solutions have a lower osmolality than plasma, approximately 250 mEq/liter
1. Infusion of hypotonic solutions may cause hypo-osmolality because these solutions have a lower concentration of electrolytes than does plasma

2. Hypotonic fluids transcend all membranes from vascular space to tissue to cell
3. Water intoxication is a serious potential complication of excessive hypotonic fluid administration
4. Examples of hypotonic solutions include 0.45% sodium chloride and 0.33% sodium chloride

J. *Hypertonic* solutions have a higher osmolality than plasma, usually greater than 375 mEq/liter
   1. Infusion of hypertonic solutions can raise plasma osmolality significantly
   2. Hypertonic fluid administration can cause vascular volume expansion and ICF deficit
   3. Complications of excessive administration of hypertonic solutions include excessive vascular volume and potential for pulmonary edema and heart failure
   4. Examples of hypertonic solutions include whole blood, albumin, total parenteral nutrition (TPN), concentrated dextrose solution (10% and greater), fat emulsions, elemental oral diets, and tube feedings

K. Nursing implications for administering oral fluid and electrolyte replacement therapy include the following:
   1. Work with the physician to calculate the patient's daily fluid requirements
   2. Using a standard chart, calculate the patient's total body surface area to accurately determine fluid needs
   3. To meet the patient's daily fluid needs, administer 1,500 ml of water for each square meter of body surface area
   4. Position the patient in semi- or high-Fowler's position to ensure safe ingestion of fluids and to avoid aspiration
   5. Check the temperature of oral fluids before administration to prevent oral mucosa burns and to promote ingestion
   6. Prepare foods and fluids as necessary, such as mixing replacement fluid with table foods, and provide portions compatible with appetite
   7. Provide a relaxed, pleasant environment to enhance the patient's appetite and promote compliance with therapy
   8. Maintain accurate fluid intake and output records
   9. Obtain the patient's daily weight, and correlate any weight gain or loss with the 24-hour total on the fluid intake and output record
   10. Increase the amount of fluid replacement to 2,400 ml/m² of body surface area for moderate fluid losses and to 3,000 ml/m² for severe fluid losses
   11. Assess the effectiveness of fluid replacement therapy by monitoring urine output, serum sodium (Na) levels, blood urea nitrogen (BUN) levels, and serum osmolality; see Appendix F, Standard I.V. Solutions Used for Fluid and Electrolyte Replacement

L. Nursing implications for administering NG tube feedings include the
   following:
   1. Constitute tube feedings as ordered or use preconstituted liquid tube
      feedings to prevent administration of hypertonic fluids
   2. Position the patient in semi-Fowler's or upright position to prevent
      aspiration
   3. Remember that intubated patients should have the endotracheal tube
      cuff inflated during feedings
   4. Before administering the feeding, check NG tube placement by
      injecting air into the tube and auscultating the stomach for a gurgling
      sound
      a. This step is not necessary for gastric and jejunostomy tubes, which
         are surgically positioned
      b. Tube placement can be verified most safely by X-ray or by checking
         the pH of aspirated gastric fluid (4.0 or less)
   5. Check for retention of formula by withdrawing aspirant; volume
      greater than 160 ml indicates retention
   6. Make sure that feedings are at room temperature to prevent
      abdominal cramping on administration
   7. Wean the patient gradually onto hypertonic tube feeding; start
      hypertonic feedings with small diluted amounts, approximately 50 to
      60 ml per feeding, in an effort to prevent diarrhea; isotonic tube
      feedings may be started at full strength
   8. Administer adequate amounts of water via the parenteral route when
      necessary to meet total fluid needs
   9. Consider using a mechanical feeding pump for continuous infusion to
      prevent possible fluid overload
   10. Use clean equipment and technique – especially for gastrostomy and
       jejunostomy tubes, which carry a high infection risk because the
       peritoneum is entered

M. Nursing implications for administering PARENTERAL FLUID and electrolyte
   replacement therapy include the following:
   1. Assess veins, degree of limb mobility, and type of fluid ordered for
      infusion to determine the optimal site for parenteral line placement
   2. Use appropriate equipment for each specific purpose, for example, a
      butterfly needle for temporary infusions and an intracatheter for long-
      term therapy or for infusion of irritating solutions or medications
   3. Label and time-tape the bottle or bag to ensure proper administration
      rate
   4. Apply a dressing at the insertion site after stabilizing the needle with
      tape to prevent infection; follow with an arm board to immobilize the
      arm
   5. Calculate and adjust the flow rate, as ordered, to prevent fluid overload
   6. Change dressings according to institutional protocol; assess the
      insertion site for redness, tenderness, and swelling

7. Infuse hypertonic solution cautiously; rapid infusion could precipitate heart failure; use of an infusion control pump is recommended
8. Administer protein infusions after 3 to 4 days of carbohydrate infusion; the daily protein requirement for adults is 1 g/kg of body weight and for children is 1 to 2 g/kg of body weight
9. Assess the compatibility of all medications with the type of fluid being administered to prevent complications; for example, dextrose 5% in water (D_5W) and dilantin are incompatible
10. Consider vitamin administration after 3 days of parenteral therapy to prevent possible vitamin deficiencies

II. Water

A. General information
1. Most water is ingested orally and directly
2. Water also can be ingested indirectly through consumption of fruits, vegetables, and meats

B. Uses: replace pure water losses

C. Administration routes
1. Oral route
2. NG route

D. Nursing implications
1. Keep in mind that nursing implications are similar to those for oral fluid and electrolyte replacement therapy (see Section I-K of this chapter)
2. Be aware that many fluid imbalances have an iatrogenic origin

III. Crystalloids

A. General information
1. CRYSTALLOID solutions are used primarily for hydration and replacement therapy
2. Crystalloid solutions are composed mainly of water with dissolved electrolytes or dextrose
3. Crystalloid solutions can be isotonic, hypertonic, or hypotonic
4. Isotonic crystalloids include D_5W, 0.9% sodium chloride, and lactated Ringer's solution
5. Hypertonic crystalloids include dextrose 10% in water and dextrose 50% in water
6. Hypotonic crystalloids include 0.45% sodium chloride and 0.25% sodium chloride

B. Composition
1. Water is included in crystalloid solutions
2. Carbohydrate solutions contain dextrose in 5% to 50% concentrations

    3. Electrolyte solutions can include Na, chloride (Cl), and other electrolytes

    4. Acid-base components include acetate, lactate, or ammonium chloride

C. Types

    1. D_5W (50 g of dextrose and water)

    2. 0.9% sodium chloride (water, 154 mEq/liter of Na, and 154 mEq/liter of Cl)

    3. Dextrose 5% and 0.45% sodium chloride (water, dextrose, 77 mEq/liter of Na, and 77 mEq/liter Cl)

    4. Dextrose 5% and 0.25% sodium chloride (water, dextrose, 34 mEq/liter of Na, and 34 mEq/liter of Cl)

    5. Ringer's solution (water and a range of electrolytes, including 130 mEq/liter of Na, 109 mEq/liter of Cl, 4 mEq/liter of K, and 3 mEq/liter of Ca)

    6. Lactated Ringer's solution (water and all the electrolytes listed for Ringer's solution plus 28 mEq/liter of lactate)

D. Uses

    1. Provide hydration

    2. Provide calories

    3. Protect protein from being used as a source of energy (D_5W)

    4. Correct Na and Cl deficits (0.9% sodium chloride)

    5. Replace ECF losses (0.9% sodium chloride)

    6. Correct acidosis (lactated Ringer's solution)

E. Administration routes

    1. I.V. infusion

    2. I.V. bolus

F. Nursing implications

    1. Keep in mind that nursing implications are similar to those for parenteral fluid replacement therapy (see Section I-M of this chapter)

    2. Administer 0.9% sodium chloride to correct Na or Cl deficits

IV. Nutritional supplements: enteral

A. General information

    1. Nutritional supplements are administered to restore or maintain a patient's nutritional status

    2. These supplements contain essential nutrients, such as amino acids, calories, electrolytes, and vitamins

B. Composition

    1. Elemental diets are a combination of water and a powdered mixture of essential and nonessential amino acids, fatty acids, glucose, electrolytes, and minerals

2. Tube feedings are a liquid mixture of water, protein, carbohydrates, fats, minerals, and vitamins; this mixture can be commercially prepared or can be liquefied whole foods

C. Types
1. Hyperosmolar elemental diets, such as Vivonex
2. Hyperosmolar tube feedings, such as Ensure and Sustacal
3. Iso-osmolar tube feedings, such as Osmolite and Isocal

D. Uses
1. Provide a caloric supplement
2. Restore and maintain nutritional status
3. Provide an additional energy source

E. Administration routes
1. Oral route
2. NG route
3. Gastric route through gastrostomy or jejunostomy tube

F. Nursing implications
1. Keep in mind that nursing implications are similar to those for oral and NG tube feedings (see Sections I-K and I-L of this chapter)
2. Dehydration due to inadequate dilution or water supplementation is a risk, especially in geriatric patients
3. Aspiration of tube feedings is a major complication

V. Nutritional supplements: parenteral

A. General information
1. Parenteral nutritional supplements are administered to restore or maintain a patient's nutritional status
2. They contain essential nutrients, such as amino acids, caloric sources, electrolytes, and often vitamins
3. Parenteral supplements are administered through a peripheral or central I.V. line
4. TPN provides a concentrated source of calories (approximately 1,000 calories/liter), as well as total nutrient requirements; TPN is administered through a central I.V. line
5. Approximately 400 calories/day must be administered in order to protect protein; a total of 1,600 calories per day are required to meet daily adult energy needs
6. Protein requirements for adults average 1 g/kg of body weight; for children, 1 to 2 g/kg
7. Ethyl alcohol provides a rich source of calories; 1 g of alcohol yields approximately 7 calories
8. Alcohol solutions usually are administered with D_5W

B. Composition
   1. Carbohydrate parenteral nutrients are composed of carbohydrates available as dextrose solutions in concentrations of 5 to 50 percent
   2. Protein parenteral solutions are composed of crystalline amino acids or colloidal elements
   3. Fat emulsions are composed of lipids in 10% and 20% concentrations
   4. TPN is composed of dextrose (25% to 50%), amino acids, and selected amounts of K, Na, calcium, phosphorus, and magnesium; water and fat-soluble vitamins also may be included
   5. Alcohol solutions contain ethyl alcohol, a rich source of calories
   6. Vitamins may include both fat-soluble and water-soluble vitamins

C. Types
   1. Crystalline amino acids or albumin-type products
   2. Fat emulsions
   3. Ethyl alcohol solutions
   4. Vitamin C, vitamin B-complex, or fat-soluble vitamins

D. Uses
   1. Provide calories
   2. Restore and maintain nutritional status
   3. Protect protein (if 400 calories/day are administered)
   4. Provide an additional energy source

E. Administration route: I.V. infusion

F. Nursing implications
   1. Keep in mind that nursing implications are similar to those for parenteral fluid replacement therapy (see Section I-M of this chapter)
   2. Be aware that fat emulsions are incompatible with electrolyte and most other solutions
   3. Do not use filters when administering fat emulsions
   4. Remember that fat emulsions are contraindicated in patients who cannot metabolize fats – for example, patients with pancreatitis
   5. When administering fat emulsions, assess for adverse reactions, such as vomiting, headache, dyspnea, allergic reaction, hyperlipidemia, temperature elevation, flushing, sweating, hepatomegaly, fat overload syndrome, and shock; also continue to monitor for delayed reactions
   6. Use a mechanical infusion pump for TPN administration because the patient is at risk for hyperosmolality with rapid infusion
   7. Infuse TPN through a central line only
   8. Assess the patient every 15 minutes during the first hour of TPN therapy to determine tolerance, then every 30 minutes thereafter
   9. Consider using a 0.22-micron filter for TPN infusion; this size inhibits passage of *Pseudomonas* bacteria and decreases the risk of contamination

10. Use meticulous sterile technique when changing TPN central line dressings; the patient is at high risk for infection because of the solution's concentrated glucose content
11. Assess laboratory studies, such as serum BUN, creatinine, and electrolyte levels, every 12 to 24 hours (or whenever the patient's condition changes) for indications of an imbalance
12. Be aware that the common imbalances associated with TPN infusion include hyperkalemia, azotemia, hypophosphatemia, metabolic acidosis, hyperglycemia, and hyperosmolar nonketotic sundrome
13. Monitor for signs and symptoms of hyperglycemia; consider the need for insulin if hyperglycemia occurs
14. Do not give fat emulsions to a patient with an allergy to eggs

VI. Colloids

A. General information
   1. A COLLOID is administered during an acute situation to expand intravascular volume and maintain blood pressure
   2. Colloids are indicated for patients with a protein deficit, such as found in starvation, liver disease, or alcohol (ETOH) abuse

B. Composition
   1. Plasma is composed of water, protein, and small amounts of carbohydrates and lipids
   2. Serum protein and albumin are composed of albumin and globulins

C. Types
   1. Fresh frozen plasma
   2. Albumin (Albumisol)
   3. Plasma protein fraction (Plasmanate)

D. Uses
   1. Restore serum protein levels
   2. Restore albumin levels
   3. Expand intravascular volume
   4. Correct hypotensive episodes

E. Administration routes
   1. I.V. infusion
   2. I.V. bolus

F. Nursing implications
   1. Keep in mind that nursing implications are similar to those for parenteral fluid replacement therapy (see Section I-M of this chapter)
   2. Be aware that colloid administration can greatly expand intravascular volume, putting the patient at risk for congestive heart failure and pulmonary edema
   3. Assess the patient's response to colloid administration by monitoring blood pressure, pulse, and central venous pressure readings

4. Monitor serum protein and albumin levels for deficits during colloid administration

VII. Blood and blood products

A. General information
   1. Normal adult blood volume averages about 75 ml/kg of body weight
   2. A plasma volume deficit of 15% to 20% is associated with hypovolemic shock

B. Types
   1. Whole blood
   2. Packed red blood cells (RBCs)
   3. Plasma
   4. Platelets
   5. Cryoprecipitate
   6. Albumin
   7. Plasma protein fraction

C. Composition
   1. Whole blood has a volume of 500 ml and contains erythrocytes and all coagulation factors except VIII and V, but lacks platelets
   2. Packed RBCs have a volume of 250 to 300 ml and contain erythrocytes and 100 ml plasma
   3. Plasma has a plasma volume of 200 to 250 ml and contains all coagulation factors, but lacks platelets (a colloid)
   4. Platelets have a plasma volume of 50 ml and contain platelets
   5. Cryoprecipitate has a plasma volume of 10 to 25 ml and contains factor VIII and fibrinogen
   6. Albumin has a volume of 50 (25 percent) to 250 (5 percent) ml and contains human albumin; it carries virtually no risk of hepatitis or human immunodeficiency virus (HIV) because of a heat treatment process used during manufacturing
   7. Plasma protein fraction is 5% albumin and globulin solution in normal saline; it carries virtually no risk of hepatitis or HIV because of a heat treatment process used during manufacturing

D. Uses
   1. Replace blood loss
   2. Replace RBC loss
   3. Treat anemia
   4. Expand blood volume

E. Administration routes: I.V. infusion

F. Nursing implications
   1. Use principles of infection control when handling blood and blood products
   2. Use a blood filter when administering blood or blood products

3. Inspect the blood bag's contents for discoloration
4. Before administration, check blood identification information against patient information, following institutional protocol
5. Assess blood temperature before administering, and use blood-warming equipment when necessary
6. Take and record baseline vital signs before blood administration, including temperature, pulse, blood pressure, and respirations
7. Adjust infusion rate to avoid the danger of bacterial growth and RBC hemolysis from infusion hanging too long; the maximum infusion time is 4 hours; use an infusion pump to regulate the flow rate according to institutional protocol
8. Monitor the patient's response to blood or blood product infusion throughout the first 15 minutes of infusion, then every 20 to 30 minutes
9. Assess for signs and symptoms of blood transfusion reaction, such as fever, chills, shortness of breath, headache, and hematuria
   a. If reactions occur, stop the infusion immediately and infuse normal saline solution to keep the vein open, using a new administration set
   b. Take the patient's vital signs
   c. Notify the physician
   d. Follow institution policies for further actions
10. Monitor for signs and symptoms of anaphylactic reaction, including respiratory distress, hypotension, rash, flushing, chills, and pruritus
11. Watch for possible complications of massive transfusion, such as hyperkalemia, acidosis, hypothermia, citrate toxicity, and 2,3-diphosphoglycerate deficiency; see Appendix G, Blood Component Therapy

Points to remember

Replacement fluids are available in three concentrations: isotonic, hypotonic, and hypertonic.

Colloids are used to expand vascular volume.

Too-rapid administration of hypertonic I.V. fluids can cause rapid vascular volume expansion and intracellular fluid (ICF) deficit, leading to pulmonary edema.

Significant blood loss is replaced with blood products.

Safety measures must be taken when blood products are administered.

Glossary

The following terms are defined in Appendix A, page 127.

colloid

crystalloid

gastrostomy

parenteral fluid

Study questions

To evaluate your understanding of this chapter, answer the following questions in the space provided; then compare your responses with the correct answers in Appendix B, pages 133 and 134.

1. What type of fluid has the same osmolality as plasma? _____

_____

_____

2. When would crystalloid solutions be used? _____

_____

_____

3. What must the nurse do before administering an NG tube feeding?

_____

_____

4. What are the safest ways of determining feeding tube placement? _____

_____

_____

5. How should TPN be administered? _____

_____

_____

6. When are colloids administered? _____

_____

7. What should the nurse do if a transfusion reaction occurs? _____

_____

_____

CHAPTER 9

Conditions Associated with Fluid, Electrolyte, and Acid-Base Imbalances

Learning objectives

Check off the following items once you've mastered them:

☐ Identify common conditions associated with fluid, electrolyte, and acid-base imbalances.

☐ Describe the specific imbalances involved in each of these conditions.

☐ Discuss how the pathophysiology of these conditions leads to imbalances.

☐ Discuss specific nursing implications for the imbalances occurring with each condition.

I. Introduction

A. Various conditions—particularly those affecting major regulatory systems—commonly result in fluid, electrolyte, or acid-base imbalances

B. Various conditions can disrupt the regulatory mechanism or action of an organ or system

C. Treatment instituted to correct a condition also can cause imbalances

D. Conditions involving excessive gains or losses of fluid, such as occurs in diuretic therapy, nasogastric suctioning, vomiting, or diarrhea, or after massive tissue destruction (for example, in burns and trauma), will result in fluid, electrolyte, and acid-base imbalances

E. Imbalances commonly result from the following:
   1. Dietary restrictions
   2. Electrolyte replacement therapy
   3. Hormonal therapy (steroids)

II. Renal failure

A. General information
   1. The renal system is a major regulator of fluid, electrolyte, and acid-base balance
   2. Renal failure involves disruption of normal kidney function; it is classified as acute renal failure (ARF) or chronic renal failure (CRF)
   3. Both ARF and CRF affect the kidneys' functional unit, the nephron
   4. ARF occurs suddenly and is usually reversible; CRF occurs slowly and insidiously and is irreversible
   5. Imbalances occur as the kidneys lose the ability to excrete water (H_2O), electrolytes, wastes, and acid-base products via the urine
   6. Patients with renal failure are at risk for fluid volume, electrolyte, and metabolic acid-base imbalances
   7. Other problems caused by renal failure that alter homeostasis include anemia, hypertension, uremia, and osteodystrophy

B. Pathophysiology
   1. The kidneys do not receive adequate blood flow because of diminished renal perfusion, either partial or complete bilateral obstruction, or nephron damage
   2. As a result, the kidneys cannot produce normal amounts of urine
   3. With abnormal urine production, the kidneys' ability to maintain homeostasis is altered

C. Potential imbalance: Extracellular fluid (ECF) volume excess
   1. H_2O and sodium (Na) retention during renal failure is associated with oliguria or anuria when the body cannot excrete excess fluid and electrolytes

2. This state can result in hypertension, peripheral edema, or pulmonary edema

D. Potential imbalance: ECF volume deficit
   1. H_2O losses in renal failure are associated with a diuretic or polyuric phase of ARF
   2. Dehydration occurs during the diuretic phase only when the large volume of urine output is not matched by adequate fluid replacement
   3. This state can result in hypotension and circulatory collapse

E. Potential imbalance: Hyperkalemia
   1. Hyperkalemia usually occurs with oliguria and anuria because potassium (K) excretion is reduced as urine output is diminished
   2. In CRF, the patient tends to tolerate high K levels; symptoms may not appear until the K level exceeds 7.5 mEq/liter
   3. In ARF, symptoms appear much earlier, often with K levels of 6 mEq/liter

F. Potential imbalance: Hypocalcemia
   1. The patient with hypocalcemia is at high risk for tetany and seizures; secondary hyperparathyroidism occurs after repeated episodes of significant hypocalcemia have caused the parathyroid gland to hypertrophy
   2. The overactive, enlarged parathyroid gland mobilizes calcium (Ca) from bone to replenish the hypocalcemic serum
   3. Bone softening—known as osteomalacia or renal rickets—occurs in the patient with repeated episodes of hypocalcemia

G. Potential imbalance: Hyperphosphatemia
   1. Hyperphosphatemia results because the kidneys lose the ability to excrete phosphate
   2. It typically occurs in CRF when the glomerular filtration rate drops below 25 to 30 ml/minute

H. Potential imbalance: Hypermagnesemia
   1. Hypermagnesemia usually occurs secondary to abuse of magnesium-containing agents, such as laxatives (MOM) and antacids
   2. Hypermagnesemia should be suspected if the patient demonstrates sudden changes in neurologic status

I. Potential imbalance: Hypernatremia
   1. Hypernatremia is less common than other imbalances
   2. It results from excessive Na retention

J. Potential imbalance: Metabolic acidosis
   1. Metabolic acidosis occurs commonly in ARF and CRF
   2. It develops as the kidneys lose the ability to secrete hydrogen (H) ions (an acid) in the urine

K. Potential imbalance: Metabolic alkalosis
   1. Metabolic alkalosis rarely occurs in renal failure
   2. It usually occurs only after excessive administration of bicarbonate in an effort to correct metabolic acidosis

L. Nursing implications
   1. Assess the patient carefully to determine the type and extent of fluid, electrolyte, or acid-base imbalance
   2. Maintain an accurate fluid intake and output record; calculate insensible H_2O losses to determine fluid balance
   3. Obtain daily weight and correlate results with the 24-hour intake and output record
   4. Monitor vital signs, including lung sounds and central venous pressure when available, to detect fluid abnormalities; report hypertension that may occur secondary to fluid and Na retention
   5. Observe for signs and symptoms of fluid overload, such as edema, bounding pulse, and shortness of breath
   6. Monitor serum electrolyte levels for abnormalities
   7. Observe for signs and symptoms that may indicate electrolyte imbalance, such as tetany, paresthesia, and muscle weakness
   8. Monitor ECG readings to detect changes secondary to hypokalemia, hyperkalemia, hypocalcemia, hypercalcemia, hypomagnesemia, and hypermagnesemia
   9. As necessary, restrict electrolyte intake, especially K and P, to prevent further imbalances
   10. Monitor arterial blood gas (ABG) studies for pH; observe for symptomatic acidosis
   11. As ordered, administer diuretics to patients whose kidneys can still respond to remove fluid excess; glomerular filtration rate should be at least 25 ml
   12. As ordered, administer medications such as oral electrolyte replacements and cation exchange resins to correct electrolyte imbalances (see Chapter 6 for specific interventions)
   13. Expect to administer sodium bicarbonate ($NaHCO_3$) intravenously to control acute acidosis and orally to control chronic acidosis
   14. Be aware of the high Na content in a dose of $NaHCO_3$ (approximately 50 mEq in one 50-ml ampule); multiple doses may result in significant hypernatremia, which could contribute to the onset of heart failure and pulmonary edema
   15. Teach the patient and family how to calculate and record amounts (in milliliters) of fluid ingested and excreted
   16. Teach the patient and family about electrolyte content in solid foods, fluids, and medications — especially over-the-counter antacids and laxatives — to prevent ingestion of excessive electrolytes

17. Be prepared to initiate dialysis for electrolyte and acid-base imbalances that do not respond to medication therapy, or when fluid removal is not possible
18. Determine the optimal "dry weight" for the dialysis patient; dry weight is individualized for each patient and obtained after dialysis

III. Congestive heart failure

A. General information
   1. In congestive heart failure (CHF), the heart cannot pump sufficient blood volume to meet the body's metabolic demands
   2. CHF may result from conditions within or affecting the heart itself (such as cardiomyopathy, atherosclerotic heart disease, or acute myocardial infarction), from inadequate venous return (as in chronic obstructive pulmonary disease (COPD) and pulmonary hypertension), from circulatory overload (such as in excessive vascular volume expansion), or from albumin or mannitol infusion
   3. In left-sided CHF, the left ventricle cannot propel the blood volume forward into the aorta; blood backs up in the pulmonary vascular bed, increasing pulmonary capillary pressure and resulting in pulmonary venous congestion
   4. In right-sided CHF, the right ventricle has difficulty propelling the blood forward into the pulmonary circulation; blood backs up into the systemic circulation, causing blood pooling in the liver and increased pressure in the peripheral circulation, resulting in edema
   5. Patients with CHF are at risk for fluid volume, electrolyte, and metabolic acid-base imbalances
   6. Imbalances may result from the heart's failure to pump and to adequately perfuse the tissues, from stimulation of the RENIN-ANGIOTENSIN-ALDOSTERONE MECHANISM, or from treatment interventions, such as diuretics

B. Pathophysiology
   1. The failing heart cannot generate the energy necessary to propel the ventricular blood volume forward
   2. Blood backs up in the system
   3. Cardiac output and hydrostatic pressure in the vascular space fall, which is reflected in a drop in blood pressure
   4. The kidneys, sensitive to the renal hypoperfusion state resulting from decreased cardiac output, trigger the renin-angiotensin-aldosterone mechanism
   5. Angiotensin II, produced from the conversion of renin and angiotensin I, acts directly on the vessels to produce a massive peripheral vasoconstriction and also stimulates the release of aldosterone, which enhances Na reabsorption at the nephron level
   6. Cardiac muscle pumping against a vasoconstricted vessel results in an increased work load (increased afterload) and exacerbates failure

7. The Na reabsorption is accompanied by H_2O reabsorption; these mechanisms cause an increased vascular volume, which compounds the existing cardiac compromise

C. Potential imbalance: ECF volume excess
   1. ECF volume excess is the most common fluid imbalance associated with CHF
   2. It results from the heart's failure to propel blood forward and consequent vascular pooling and from the Na and H_2O reabsorption triggered by the renin mechanism
   3. ECF volume excess commonly causes peripheral edema

D. Potential imbalance: ECF volume deficit usually associated with overaggressive diuretic therapy

E. Potential imbalance: Hypokalemia
   1. Hypokalemia is caused by prolonged diuretic use without adequate K replacement
   2. Hypokalemia potentiates digitalis toxicity if the patient is receiving digitalis

F. Potential imbalance: Hyponatremia
   1. Hyponatremia may result from Na loss because of diuretic abuse
   2. In some cases, hyponatremia may result from a dilutional effect caused by greater H_2O reabsorption than Na reabsorption

G. Potential imbalance: Hypernatremia
   1. Hypernatremia may occur if diuretic use produces much greater H_2O loss than Na loss
   2. It also may be linked to an overactive renin mechanism causing excessive Na reabsorption

H. Potential imbalance: Hypochloremia resulting from excessive diuretic therapy

I. Potential imbalance: Metabolic acidosis
   1. Metabolic acidosis is linked to excessive lactic acid production
   2. The lactic acid buildup results from significantly reduced tissue perfusion in a compromised individual

J. Potential imbalance: Metabolic alkalosis resulting from excessive diuretic use leading to secretion of hydrochloric acid (HCl)

K. Nursing implications
   1. Monitor Na and H_2O intake, as ordered, because hyponatremia and fluid volume deficit can stimulate the renin-angiotensin-aldosterone mechanism and exacerbate CHF; usually, a mild Na restriction — such as no added salt — with no H_2O restriction is implemented
   2. Monitor fluid status; check daily weight and fluid intake and output for significant changes

3. Monitor vital signs, including blood pressure, pulse, respirations, and lung sounds for abnormalities that might indicate a fluid excess or deficit
4. Assess for signs and symptoms of impending cardiac failure, such as fatigue; restlessness; rapid, thready pulse; hypotension; decreased heart sounds; murmurs; gallop rhythms; rapid respirations; dyspnea; coughing; decreased urine output; and liver enlargement
5. Assess for the presence, amount, and location of edema; note the presence and degree of any pitting
6. Monitor serum electrolyte levels, such as Na and K, for changes that may indicate an imbalance
7. As ordered, administer medications, such as digoxin, diuretics, and K supplements, to support cardiac function and minimize symptoms
8. Administer oral K supplements in orange juice or with meals to promote absorption and prevent gastric irritation

IV. Respiratory insufficiency

A. General information
   1. The lungs are a major regulator of fluid, electrolyte, and acid-base balance
   2. In respiratory insufficiency, the lungs cannot maintain adequate gas exchange
   3. Respiratory insufficiency may result from hypoxemia secondary to increased pulmonary capillary pressure or permeability (for example, in left-sided CHF or pneumonia); from conditions impairing normal carbon dioxide (CO_2) elimination (such as COPD or asthmatic crisis); or from neuromuscular impairment of respiratory drive (such as can occur in drug overdoses, spinal cord injury, multiple sclerosis, or myasthenia gravis)
   4. Patients with respiratory insufficiency are at risk for fluid volume, electrolyte, and respiratory acid-base imbalances
   5. Imbalances result from ventilatory impairment, which leads to excessive CO_2 retention or elimination or to excessive fluid losses through the lungs

B. Pathophysiology
   1. Inadequate oxygenation results in hypoxemia, leading to hypocapnia and an increased respiratory rate
   2. An increased respiratory rate leads to increased insensible fluid loss through the lungs and excessive elimination of CO_2
   3. Insufficient respiratory center stimulation results in hypercapnia, leading to hypoxemia
   4. Airway obstruction results in CO_2 retention and hypercapnia, limiting the amount of CO_2 eliminated by the lungs; respiratory rate may be normal or increased

C. Potential imbalance: Respiratory acidosis
1. Respiratory acidosis results from the lungs' inability to eliminate adequate amounts of CO_2
2. Excessive CO_2 combines with H_2O to form carbonic acid (H_22CO_3)
3. Increased H_2CO_3 levels result in decreased pH, contributing to respiratory acidosis

D. Potential imbalance: Respiratory alkalosis
1. Respiratory alkalosis results from too-rapid respirations, causing excessive CO_2 elimination
2. The loss of CO_2 decreases the serum's acid-forming potential, resulting in respiratory alkalosis

E. Potential imbalance: ECF volume excess
1. Prolonged respiratory treatment, such as nebulizers, can lead to the inhalation of H_2O vapor and its absorption through lung tissue; excessive fluid absorption may also result from increased pulmonary capillary pressure or permeability
2. This excessive fluid absorption can precipitate pulmonary edema

F. Potential imbalance: ECF volume deficit
1. H_2O as vapor normally is eliminated during respiration
2. Excessive H_2O loss occurs in fever or any condition that increases the metabolic rate and thus the respiratory rate

G. Nursing implications
1. Monitor ABG levels to assess oxygenation and pH status
2. Assess lung status; monitor rate, depth, and character of respirations, making sure to check lung sounds for abnormalities
3. Administer oxygen as ordered to help maintain adequate oxygenation and restore the normal respiratory rate
4. Administer oxygen to the patient with COPD cautiously because adequate serum oxygen levels depress the stimulus for breathing
5. Perform chest physiotherapy and postural drainage as needed to promote adequate ventilation
6. As necessary, intervene to correct the underlying respiratory problem and respiratory-based alterations in acid-base status
7. Monitor fluid status by maintaining accurate fluid intake and output records
8. Evaluate serum electrolyte levels for abnormalities that can occur with acid-base imbalances

V. Burns

A. General information
1. A burn refers to the destruction of the epidermis, dermis, or subcutaneous layers of the skin that can result from radiation; mechanical injury, such as friction; chemicals; electrical injury, such as lightning or electrical wires; or thermal injury, such as fire or frostbite

2. Imbalances associated with burns result from alterations in skin integrity and internal body membranes and from the effect of heat on body H_2O and solute losses that result from cellular destruction

3. The type and severity of the imbalance depend on the burn type and depth, the percentage of body surface area involved, and the burn phase

4. The percentage of body surface area involved is determined by the "rule of nines" – the greater the body surface involved, the greater the potential for imbalances

5. Burn depth is classified as first-, second-, or third-degree

6. *First-degree burns* (superficial partial thickness) involve superficial injury to the epidermis marked by an uncomplicated erythematous area; because the skin barrier remains intact, fluid loss is not a problem

7. *Second-degree burns* (dermal partial thickness) involve damage to the epidermis, progressing to the dermis; blisters are present, and capillary damage is possible; regeneration of the epithelial layer may occur

8. *Third-degree burns* (full thickness) involve all skin layers; regeneration is not possible; skin appearance is altered significantly and elasticity is lost; skin color varies from red to black to white

9. Third-degree burns carry the greatest risk of imbalances

10. Burn phases refer to the stages that describe physiologic changes that occur after a burn; they include the fluid accumulation phase, fluid remobilization phase, and the convalescent phase

B. Pathophysiology
    1. About 10% of plasma volume is lost into the tissue early after a severe burn because of edema caused by increased capillary permeability
    2. Further extravasation into areas other than the tissue, such as cells and third spaces, accounts for losses, sometimes greater than 40%; evaporation of H_2O secondary to the heat loss from skin destruction results in an even greater volume loss, accounting for as much as 4 liters/day
    3. Intravascular H_2O is rich in serum proteins, electrolytes, and essential minerals; damaged capillaries at the burn site leak their fluid into the interstitial space, resulting in solute deficits
    4. Decreased tissue perfusion precipitates lactic acid formation
    5. Diminished respiratory excursion may cause CO_2 retention
    6. Disruption of the natural skin barrier promotes fluid losses and also increases the risk of infection

C. Potential imbalance: ECF volume excess
    1. ECF volume excess usually develops 3 to 5 days after a major burn injury
    2. It occurs as fluid shifts from the interstitial space back to plasma

D. Potential imbalance: ECF volume deficit
  1. In burns, ECF volume deficit involves both extravasated fluid and fluid losses
  2. Composition of fluid losses resembles intravascular fluid that contains proteins and serum electrolytes
  3. Blood loss also may occur, adding to fluid volume losses

E. Potential imbalance: Hyperkalemia
  1. In burns, hyperkalemia results from massive cellular trauma, metabolic acidosis, or renal failure
  2. Hyperkalemia develops as K is released into the ECF during the fluid accumulation phase

F. Potential imbalance: Hypokalemia
  1. In burns, hypokalemia develops as K shifts from the ECF into the cells
  2. Hypokalemia usually occurs 4 to 5 days after a major burn injury

G. Potential imbalance: Hypocalcemia
  1. Hypocalcemia can develop in burns as Ca travels to the damaged tissue and becomes immobilized at the burn site
  2. Hypocalcemia may occur 12 to 24 hours after the burn

H. Potential imbalance: Hyponatremia
  1. Hyponatremia results from increased intracellular H_2O and Na losses
  2. Large amounts of Na are trapped in edema fluid and burn exudate
  3. Na is also lost when diuresis occurs during the fluid remobilization phase

I. Potential imbalance: Metabolic acidosis
  1. Tissue perfusion becomes ineffective because of intravascular fluid shifts and overall fluid losses
  2. Fixed acids released from injured tissues accumulate, causing a drop in pH

J. Potential imbalance: Respiratory acidosis secondary to inadequate ventilation

K. Nursing implications
  1. As ordered, administer intravenous (I.V.) fluid therapy to restore depleted vascular volume; lactated Ringer's solution is usually the solution of choice
  2. Calculate the amount of fluid replacement necessary; infuse 50% of this volume in the first 8 hours postburn and the remainder over the next 16 hours, as ordered
  3. Do not administer colloid solutions in the immediate postburn period; colloids will increase osmotic pressure in the interstitial space, which may exacerbate burn edema and increase the risk of vascular collapse

4. Remember that maintenance I.V. fluid replacement is based on daily assessment of fluid, electrolyte, acid-base, and nutritional needs
5. Administer I.V. electrolyte replacement therapy as ordered during the initial postburn period; monitor for signs and symptoms of hypokalemia, hyponatremia, and hypocalcemia
6. Use the oral route for electrolyte replacement as soon as patients can tolerate it; patients usually experience a paralytic ileus after burns
7. Assess for signs and symptoms of metabolic acidosis and possibly respiratory acidosis secondary to impaired ventilation
8. Provide oxygen therapy as ordered to promote optimal respiratory function; consider mechanical ventilation for a patient with inadequate ventilation for any reason, especially smoke inhalation
9. Promote respiratory airway excursion to ensure adequate gas exchange
10. Maintain blood pressure within the normal range to ensure adequate tissue perfusion and to prevent lactic acid production
11. Assess for upper airway obstruction secondary to smoke inhalation; monitor for its signs and symptoms, such as tachypnea, hoarseness, wheezing, and stridor
12. Assess skin for location, depth, and extent of burn
13. Assess cardiac and hemodynamic status for changes that indicate fluid imbalance
14. Monitor ECG readings for changes pointing to fluid and electrolyte imbalances, especially K imbalances
15. Assess fluid and hydration status, including skin turgor, daily weight, and hourly urine output, for significant changes
16. Monitor ABG values and serum electrolyte levels to detect any significant changes
17. Assess the patient's nutritional status; total parenteral nutrition (TPN) may be necessary to meet the patient's increased metabolic needs
18. Perform burn care as ordered; monitor the patient's response
19. Observe the patient for signs and symptoms of infection, such as fever, tachycardia, and purulent wound drainage, because the patient has an increased risk of infection exacerbated by destruction of the skin barrier and nutrient losses

VI. Diabetic ketoacidosis

A. General information
1. Diabetic ketoacidosis (DKA) is an acute condition resulting from insulin deficiency in a patient with insulin-dependent diabetes
2. In DKA, insufficient insulin is available to metabolize glucose; this condition may result from the patient's failure to take the prescribed insulin dose or from additional stressors, such as infection, trauma, or surgery

    3. DKA is characterized by hyperglycemia, ketonuria, hyperosmolality, ketonemia, and acidosis (see *Comparing DKA and HNKS*, pages 114 and 115)

    4. Imbalances occur primarily as a result of hyperglycemia

B. Pathophysiology

    1. Insufficient insulin results in an inability to metabolize glucose, as reflected by elevated serum glucose levels (exceeding 200 mg/dl)

    2. Fats are then burned for energy, resulting in ketosis (ketones are metabolic body acids)

    3. Ketone bodies accumulate in ECF, and H ions are exchanged for K

    4. Large volumes of glucose in the serum create elevated serum osmolality

    5. Elevated glucose levels in the renal tubules precipitate osmotic diuresis with losses of H_2O, Na, chloride (Cl), and K

    6. Significant dehydration and electrolyte deficits follow inadequate volume replacement

    7. These deficits trigger pulmonary and renal compensatory mechanisms

    8. The lungs attempt to eliminate excess acids through deep and rapid respirations (Kussmaul respirations) to compensate for the increase in metabolic acids (ketones)

    9. The kidneys attempt to increase acid excretion in the urine (ketonuria)

C. Potential imbalance: ECF volume deficit

    1. ECF volume deficit results from osmotic diuresis

    2. Excessive H_2O is lost as the kidneys attempt to rid the body of excess acids

D. Potential imbalance: Hypokalemia

    1. Hypokalemia in DKA results from osmotic diuresis

    2. ECF volume deficit increases aldosterone secretion, which in turn leads to K loss

    3. Intracellular movement of K in response to ketone accumulation and metabolic acidosis can exacerbate the imbalance

E. Potential imbalance: Hyponatremia secondary to osmotic diuresis

F. Potential imbalance: Hypophosphatemia secondary to treatment for DKA

G. Potential imbalance: Metabolic acidosis

    1. In DKA, fats are broken down for energy into ketones

    2. Ketones (strong acids) accumulate in the blood, increasing the amount of fixed acids and thus lowering the pH

H. Nursing implications

    1. Carefully monitor serum glucose and electrolyte levels, serum osmolality, and ABG results

2. Monitor daily weight and intake and output records; insert an indwelling (Foley) catheter in a comatose patient to monitor urine output accurately
3. Administer insulin, as ordered, correlating dosage with serum glucose levels
4. Provide initial rehydration with 0.9% sodium chloride (NaCl) or lactated Ringer's solution as ordered; rapid volume replacement may necessitate a rate as rapid as 1 liter/hour
5. Be prepared to administer bicarbonate for severe acidosis that does not respond to insulin
6. Assess hemodynamic parameters to determine the amount of volume replacement necessary to maintain adequate blood pressure and urine output
7. Avoid creating a hypoglycemic state with fluid replacement therapy; a rapid change in serum osmolality can precipitate cerebral edema
8. Replace K gradually with I.V. fluids; correction of metabolic acidosis releases K from cells

VII. Hyperosmolar nonketotic syndrome

A. General information
   1. Hyperosmolar nonketotic syndrome (HNKS) is an acute condition characterized by insulin deficiency in a patient with diabetes
   2. In HNKS, some insulin is present but not enough to metabolize glucose
   3. HNKS is characterized by hyperglycemia, hyperosmolality, and osmotic diuresis; ketosis and ketonuria do not occur (see *Comparing DKA and HNKS*, pages 114 and 115)
   4. HNKS typically occurs in middle-aged or geriatric patients with the onset of diabetes; it also may develop as a severe exacerbation of previously non-insulin-dependent diabetes
   5. Imbalances associated with HNKS include fluid volume and electrolyte imbalances that result primarily from osmotic diuresis

B. Pathophysiology
   1. Insulin is present in sufficient amounts to prevent ketosis but in insufficient amounts to prevent hyperglycemia
   2. Hyperglycemia results in hyperosmolality and osmotic diuresis
   3. The urine contains relatively greater amounts of H_2O than Na

C. Potential imbalance: ECF volume deficit related to osmotic diuresis

D. Potential imbalance: Hypokalemia resulting from osmotic diuresis

E. Potential imbalance: Hypophosphatemia secondary to osmotic diuresis

F. Potential imbalance: Hypernatremia resulting from proportionately greater H_2O loss than Na loss

COMPARING D.K.A. AND H.N.K.S.

	DKA	HNKS
Parameters	Usually occurs in known Type I diabetic patients	Usually occurs in Type II diabetic patients (condition may be undiagnosed)
Precipitating factors	Undiagnosed diabetes, neglected treatment, infection, cardiovascular disorders, physical stress, emotional distress	Undiagnosed diabetes, infection or other stress, acute or chronic illnesses, certain drugs, such medical procedures as TPN or tube feedings, severe burns treated with high sugar concentrations
Symptom onset	Slow (hours to days)	Slow (hours to days) but less gradual than DKA
Signs and symptoms		
Skin and mucous membranes	Warm, flushed, dry, loose skin; dry, crusty mucous membranes; soft eyeballs	Warm, flushed, dry, extremely loose skin; dry, crusty mucous membranes; soft eyeballs
Neurologic status	*Initial*—dullness, confusion, lethargy; diminished reflexes *Late*—coma	*Initial*—dullness, confusion, lethargy, diminished reflexes *Late*—coma
Muscle strength	Extremely weak	Extremely weak
Gastrointestinal	Anorexia, nausea, vomiting, diarrhea, abdominal tenderness and pain	Nausea, vomiting, abdominal pain
Temperature	Possible fever (from dehydration or infection)	Possible fever (from dehydration)
Pulse	Mild tachycardia, weak	Usually rapid
Blood pressure	Low	Low
Respirations	*Initial*—deep, fast *Late*—Kussmaul's	Rapid (but no Kussmaul's)
Breath odor	Fruity, acetone	Normal
Weight	Decreased	Decreased
Other	Thirst	Thirst
Laboratory findings		
Blood glucose level	Above normal	Markedly above normal
Serum sodium level	Normal or subnormal	Above normal, normal
Serum potassium level	(Normal or above normal initially) subnormal	(Normal or above normal initially) subnormal

(continued)

COMPARING D.K.A. AND H.N.K.S. *(continued)*

	DKA	HNKS
Laboratory findings *(continued)*		
Serum ketones	Positive/large	Negative/small
Serum osmolarity	Above normal but usually less than 330 mOsm/liter	Markedly above normal— 350 to 450 mOsm/liter
Hematocrit	Above normal	Above normal
Arterial blood gases	Metabolic acidosis with compensatory respiratory alkalosis	Normal
Urine glucose level	Above normal	Markedly above normal
Urine ketones	Positive/large	Negative/small
Urine output	Initial—polyuria Late—oliguria	Markedly above normal
Treatment	Insulin, fluid replacement, electrolyte replacement, antiacidosis therapy (if needed)	Fluid replacement, insulin, electrolyte replacement

G. Nursing implications
   1. Administer hypotonic 0.9% NaCl as ordered; if volume deficit is severe, use 0.9% NaCl to expand plasma volume at the prescribed flow rate to prevent overload
   2. Assess hydration status for changes indicating imbalances by monitoring intake and output, daily weight, and skin turgor
   3. Monitor serum glucose and electrolyte levels and plasma osmolality for changes
   4. Administer insulin as ordered, adjusting insulin dosage to serum glucose levels
   5. Evaluate renal function before administering K replacement; K can be added to the I.V. fluid or given as an oral supplement
   6. Be aware that severe hypophosphatemia may be treated with potassium phosphate (K_2PO_4); carefully monitor patients receiving K_2PO_4 for hyperphosphatemia, especially a patient with diminished renal function

VIII. Syndrome of inappropriate antidiuretic hormone

A. General information
   1. Syndrome of inappropriate antidiuretic hormone (SIADH) is characterized by inappropriate secretion of antidiuretic hormone (ADH) without regard for serum osmolality

2. SIADH may result from head trauma, central nervous system disorders, pulmonary disorders, endocrine disorders, and use of certain medications, such as osmotic diuretics
3. Imbalances associated with SIADH include fluid volume and electrolyte imbalances

B. Pathophysiology
1. Secretion of ADH is continuous and inappropriate
2. Prolonged ADH secretion results in H_2O retention, which leads to serum hypo-osmolality
3. Urine osmolality is greater than serum osmolality
4. H_2O reabsorption in the tubules increases, resulting in increased intravascular fluid volume
5. The glomerular filtration rate increases, inhibiting the reabsorption of Na and H_2O
6. Increased intravascular fluid volume inhibits the release of renin and aldosterone, resulting in further urine Na losses

C. Potential imbalance: ECF volume excess
1. Tubular reabsorption of H_2O is increased because of continued ADH secretion
2. H_2O is retained, leading to increased intravascular fluid volume

D. Potential imbalance: Hyponatremia
1. Hyponatremia occurs as a result of aldosterone inhibition
2. Decreased aldosterone secretion results in further urine Na losses

E. Nursing implications
1. Maintain accurate intake and output records; monitor for fluid intake exceeding output
2. Monitor daily weight for increases; correlate weights with fluid gains or losses; a 1-lb weight gain is equal to 500 ml of fluid
3. Monitor serum Na levels for abnormalities, and assess for signs and symptoms of hyponatremia; monitor serum and urine osmolality for changes
   a. In severe hyponatremia, expect to administer I.V. hypertonic saline solution to replace Na
   b. When doing so, use a volume control device to prevent overload
4. Expect to administer a diuretic—usually furosemide—concomitantly with I.V. hypertonic saline solution to promote H_2O excretion
5. Depending on urine output, restrict daily fluid intake to approximately 500 to 700 ml; consider all intake routes when imposing fluid restrictions
6. Intervene as appropriate to treat the underlying cause of SIADH
7. Institute safety precautions to minimize risk of injury in patients with changes in sensorium

8. Be aware that the physician may order lithium or phenytoin as possible therapy; keep in mind that demeclocycline also may be used to decrease the renal response to ADH

IX. Postoperative response

A. General information
  1. The preoperative and operative phases are major stressors that trigger the physiologic stress response, which may affect fluid, electrolyte, and acid-base balance
  2. The symptoms associated with postoperative phase imbalances result from the body's stress response
  3. Resolution of this phase is marked by a diuretic phase
  4. Studying the postoperative response provides a perspective on how the body responds to other stressors
  5. Fluid volume, electrolyte, and metabolic acid-base imbalances result from surgery
  6. Surgery can cause deficiencies of all electrolytes; these deficiencies may persist if not corrected

B. Pathophysiology
  1. The SYMPATHETIC RESPONSE causes increased heart rate and contractility and vasoconstriction
  2. Adrenocorticotropic hormone stimulates the release of MINERALOCORTICOIDS and GLUCOCORTICOIDS
  3. The mineralocorticoids, primarily in the form of aldosterone, stimulate the reabsorption of Na and H_2O at the renal tubules
  4. The glucocorticoids promote the mobilization of fats and the breakdown of protein and glycogen; glucocorticoids also suppress the immune system, increasing the patient's susceptibility to infection
  5. The stress response stimulates the hypothalamus, which leads to ADH release
  6. The adrenal medulla is stimulated to release increased amounts of norepinephrine and epinephrine, leading to intense vasoconstriction
  7. Systemic vasoconstriction causes localized reduction in renal blood flow, triggering the renin-angiotensin-aldosterone mechanism and leading to further vasoconstriction and Na and H_2O retention

C. Potential imbalance: ECF volume excess
  1. In most cases of ECF volume excess, ADH, aldosterone, and renin combine to promote excessive reabsorption of Na and H_2O
  2. ECF volume excess also may result from overadministration of Na-containing fluids in the first few postoperative days

D. Potential imbalance: ECF volume deficit resulting from internal or external fluid loss associated with surgical procedure or fluid status before the procedure

E. Potential imbalance: Third-space shifting
   1. Third-space shifting results from surgery's effect on tissue injury
   2. A third space is created around the operative site
   3. Fluids move to this third space, and edema forms in and about the operative site during the first few postoperative days

F. Potential imbalance: Hypokalemia
   1. Hypokalemia can result from increased K excretion because of increased secretion of mineralocorticoids and glucocorticoids
   2. K losses secondary to a surgical procedure also contribute to hypokalemia

G. Potential imbalance: Hyponatremia
   1. Hyponatremia is common in the first or second postoperative day
   2. It commonly results from excessive ADH secretion in response to stress
   3. It also may be caused by excessive administration of I.V. fluids, such as dextrose 5% in H_2O (D_5W)

H. Potential imbalance: Respiratory acidosis
   1. Respiratory acidosis commonly results from diminished ventilation and respiratory depression because of anesthesia or narcotics
   2. It also may result from impaired oxygen exchange, such as in atelectasis or airway obstruction
   3. It also may be linked to decreased respiratory depth because of abdominal distention or postoperative pain

I. Potential imbalance: Metabolic acidosis
   1. Postoperative metabolic acidosis usually is secondary to the surgical tissue destruction, resulting in increased H ion production
   2. Reduced urine output also reduces H ion secretion
   3. Metabolic acidosis also can result from excessive losses of intestinal, bile, or pancreatic juices

J. Potential imbalance: Metabolic alkalosis
   1. Postoperative metabolic alkalosis commonly occurs in patients who have lost a large amount of gastric secretions
   2. It is closely associated with hypokalemia and hypochloremia

K. Nursing implications
   1. Anticipate the possibility of postoperative phase imbalances resulting from the physiologic aspects of the patient's stress response
   2. Promote stress reduction; provide preoperative teaching, allow family visits, keep the patient informed about recovery progress, and encourage expression of feelings and concerns
   3. Provide adequate nutrition (calories, protein, vitamins, and minerals) to counteract the catabolic effect of glucocorticoids, to replace nutrients, to promote healing, and to prevent infection

4. Assess patient progress by monitoring vital signs, intake and output, and daily weight
5. Assess wound drain sites for amount and character of drainage and record
6. Support the patient's return to a homeostatic state by promoting regular ambulation, turning, coughing, and deep breathing
7. Administer I.V. fluid replacement therapy as ordered
8. Monitor serum electrolyte levels for abnormalities

X. Intestinal obstruction

A. General information
  1. Intestinal obstruction involves interference with the normal peristaltic movement of intestinal contents
  2. Obstruction may result from a physical barrier or from impairment of bowel innervation resulting in an inability to move the digested food forward
  3. Imbalances associated with intestinal obstruction include fluid volume and metabolic acid-base imbalances

B. Pathophysiology
  1. A bowel obstruction causes hyperperistalsis and trauma to the intestinal wall
  2. Intestinal gas and fluid accumulate proximal to the obstruction
  3. Large quantities of H_2O and electrolytes are secreted into the bowel or peritoneal area and form a third space
  4. Plasma proteins enter the intestinal lumen, causing increased distention
  5. The portion of the intestines above the obstruction continues to secrete more fluid; the edematous bowel cannot absorb this large fluid volume, leading to increased distention and volume depletion

C. Potential imbalance: ECF volume deficit
  1. ECF volume deficit results from trapped fluid in the intestines, prolonged vomiting, or excessive GI suctioning
  2. Volume loss may be 5 liters or more

D. Potential imbalance: Third-space shifting
  1. The altered bowel wall contributes to the formation of an abnormal compartment
  2. Third-space shifting results from fluid accumulation in this abnormal space

E. Potential imbalance: Metabolic acidosis
  1. Metabolic acidosis may result from vomiting larger amounts of alkaline intestinal fluids than acidic gastric fluids
  2. The vomiting usually occurs from obstruction in the distal small intestines

F. Potential imbalance: Metabolic alkalosis (rare) resulting from excessive vomiting of large amounts of gastric fluid

G. Potential imbalance: Respiratory acidosis
  1. Respiratory acidosis is usually linked to marked abdominal distention
  2. This distension increases pressure on the diaphragm and impairs respiratory excursion

H. Nursing implications
  1. Administer I.V. isotonic or hypotonic solutions (usually lactated Ringer's solution or D_5W) to replace fluid losses; administer at the prescribed rate to prevent overload
  2. Remember that isotonic 0.9% NaCl may be used if gastric fluid loss is excessive
  3. Administer Na and K replacements based on the patient's serum electrolyte levels; monitor these levels closely to prevent imbalances
  4. Assess hydration status by monitoring intake and output, daily weight, and skin turgor
  5. Monitor vital signs, especially pulse rate and blood pressure, to detect changes indicating fluid imbalance
  6. Evaluate the need for TPN or alternate feeding methods to maintain or restore nutritional status
  7. Assess the presence and character of bowel sounds and stool quantity and character to detect resolution of obstruction
  8. Monitor gastrointestinal (GI) suction for amount and character of drainage
  9. Prepare the patient for possible surgical intervention

XI. Excessive GI fluid loss

A. General information
  1. GI fluid loss may include loss of saliva, gastric juices, bile, pancreatic juice, and intestinal secretions
  2. All GI fluids are isotonic—except saliva, which is hypotonic
  3. GI fluid loss is the most common cause of fluid and electrolyte imbalances
  4. GI fluids may be lost through excessive vomiting, gastric suctioning, diarrhea, intestinal suctioning, ileostomy, and fistulas

B. Pathophysiology
  1. Gastric, intestinal, and pancreatic fluids contain large amounts of Na, K, and Cl
  2. Gastric fluid is highly acidic; intestinal and pancreatic fluids and bile are alkaline
  3. Loss of gastric fluids through vomiting or gastric suctioning results in loss of acid, specifically HCl

4. Loss of intestinal and pancreatic juices and bile through diarrhea, intestinal suctioning, fistulas, and ileostomy results in loss of alkaline fluids
5. Losses of either type result in loss of Na, K, and Cl

C. Potential imbalance: ECF volume deficit
   1. ECF volume deficit can result from gastric and intestinal fluid losses
   2. Large amounts of fluid, including H_2O, can be lost if the condition causing the loss is prolonged and not corrected

D. Potential imbalance: Hypokalemia resulting from prolonged loss of gastric or intestinal fluid

E. Potential imbalance: Hyponatremia resulting from prolonged vomiting, diarrhea, or gastric or intestinal suctioning

F. Potential imbalance: Metabolic acidosis
   1. Metabolic acidosis can result from prolonged diarrhea, intestinal suctioning, or excessive ileostomy drainage
   2. Bicarbonate ions in intestinal fluids are lost in large quantities

G. Potential imbalance: Metabolic alkalosis
   1. Metabolic alkalosis can result from prolonged vomiting or gastric suctioning
   2. H and Cl in gastric fluid are lost in large amounts

H. Nursing implications
   1. Measure and record the amount of fluid lost by vomiting, suctioning, or diarrhea
   2. Assess hydration status, including intake and output, daily weight, and skin turgor; include GI losses as part of output
   3. Administer oral fluids containing H_2O and electrolytes (such as Gatorade and Pedialyte) if the patient can tolerate fluids; maintain the patient on nothing-by-mouth (NPO) status if he or she cannot tolerate fluids
   4. Administer I.V. fluids as ordered for replacement; monitor the infusion rate and volume to prevent overload
   5. Check tube placement often if the patient has gastric suctioning to prevent possible fluid aspiration
   6. Irrigate the suction tube with isotonic 0.9% NaCl as ordered; remember that plain H_2O is never used for irrigation because it may potentiate fluid and electrolyte imbalances
   7. Restrict the amount of ice chips given to the patient; too much H_2O from ice chips can cause further electrolyte imbalances
   8. As ordered, administer medications such as antiemetics or antidiarrheals to control the underlying problem
   9. Evaluate serum electrolyte levels to detect further abnormalities and to monitor the effectiveness of therapy

XII. Diuretic use

A. General information
   1. Diuretics are used to remove excess H_2O and Na from the body in edematous states, such as CHF, renal failure, and liver failure
   2. Diuretics also are indicated for the treatment of cardiovascular disease, particularly for hypertension
   3. The resulting increase in urine loss from diuretic use places the patient at risk for fluid imbalances, as well as electrolyte and acid-base imbalances
   4. The imbalances that occur result from the drug class's mechanism of action and its site of action in the kidney
   5. There are five major classes of diuretics: loop, osmotic, thiazide, K-sparing, and carbonic anhydrase inhibitors

B. Pathophysiology
   1. Diuretics remove excess H_2O and, along with it, Na from the body
   2. Loop diuretics, such as furosemide and ethacrynic acid, work primarily in the loop of Henle
      a. They block reabsorption of NaCl
      b. This reabsorption leads to diuresis of H_2O
      c. K is lost passively with the high urinary flow state
   3. Osmotic diuretics, such as mannitol, create an osmotic effect in the nephron tubule; H_2O, in response to the osmotic effect, is drawn into the tubular space and excreted in the urine
   4. Thiazide diuretics, such as hydrochlorothiazide, act on the loop of Henle
      a. They inhibit Na reabsorption
      b. K loss results along with H_2O excretion
   5. K-sparing diuretics, such as spironolactone, inhibit the action of aldosterone
      a. They enhance Na excretion; K reabsorption follows
      b. This process causes a mild diuresis but helps to preserve the body's K level
      c. Patients may receive this type of diuretic in conjunction with another more potent diuretic to prevent hypokalemia
   6. Carbonic anhydrase inhibitors, such as acetazolamide sodium, are used when an alkaline urine is desired
      a. They inhibit the action of the enzyme carbonic anhydrase, resulting in the increased secretion of $NaHCO_3$
      b. H_2O and $NaHCO_3$ are lost in the urine
      c. This loss can lead to a potential onset of metabolic acidosis
   7. Any other agent, such as digoxin, aminophylline, or dopamine, increases cardiac output; therefore, blood flow to the kidneys will contribute to the formation of a high urinary flow state or diuresis

C. Potential imbalance: Hypokalemia
1. Hypokalemia is the most common and most serious side effect of using diuretics
2. K is lost passively in the urine
3. This problem often necessitates using a K supplement, either pharmacologic or nutritional

D. Potential imbalance: Hyponatremia resulting from the action of most diuretics targeted at the enhancement of Na excretion in the urine

E. Potential imbalance: Hypochloremia
1. Hypochloremia is associated with the use of loop diuretics
2. Cl also is lost in the urine and will precipitate the onset of metabolic alkalosis
3. Use of a potassium chloride (KCl) supplement can prevent this problem

F. Potential imbalance: Hypomagnesemia
1. Hypomagnesemia is associated with the onset of hypokalemia
2. Hypomagnesemia must be corrected before the hypokalemia can be corrected to prevent further loss of K at the renal site

G. Potential imbalance: Metabolic acidosis
1. Metabolic acidosis is associated the use of carbonic anhydrase inhibitors
2. The use of carbonic anhydrase inhibitors contributes to the onset of metabolic acidosis by stimulating the excretion of $NaHCO_3$

H. Potential imbalance: Metabolic alkalosis
1. The onset of hypochloremia causes the body to compensate by stimulating the reabsorption of bicarbonate
2. The increased bicarbonate may lead to metabolic alkalosis

I. Nursing implications
1. Determine with the health care team the fluid and electrolyte goal to be reached through the use of a diuretic
2. Assess the patient closely for any signs and symptoms of a fluid, electrolyte, or acid-base imbalance
3. Monitor serum laboratory values closely, and notify the physician of any changes; check serum electrolyte levels, blood urea nitrogen (BUN), creatinine, and ABGs
4. Determine the effectiveness of the diuretic; monitor intake and output records
   a. Note if and when the patient develops a tolerance to the diuretic
   b. Keep in mind that unresponsiveness to a diuretic may be associated with a fluid and electrolyte problem
5. Monitor daily weight, and record
6. Administer diuretics in the morning
7. Teach the patient about the side effects of diuretic use
   a. Instruct the patient in signs and symptoms of imbalances
   b. Teach the patient about foods high in electrolytes

Points to remember

Renal dysfunction often leads to the retention of fluids, electrolytes, acid-base components, and wastes.

In congestive heart failure (CHF), imbalances may result from the heart's failure to pump and to adequately perfuse the tissues, from stimulation of the renin-angiotensin-aldosterone mechanism, or from treatment interventions, such as diuretics.

Imbalances linked to respiratory insufficiency result from ventilatory impairment leading to excessive carbon dioxide (CO_2) retention or elimination or fluid losses through the lungs.

Fluid loss in burns results from evaporation, heat loss, and extracellular fluid (ECF) losses secondary to increased vascular permeability.

Endocrine problems, such as diabetic ketoacidosis (DKA), hyperosmolar nonketotic syndrome (HNKS), and syndrome of inappropriate ADH secretion (SIADH), lead to numerous imbalances resulting from altered hormonal regulation.

Postoperative response is a physiologic stress response that affects the body's fluid, electrolyte, and acid-base balance.

Fluid loss from the GI tract can be alkaline (intestinal) or acidic (gastric).

Fluid, electrolyte, and acid-base imbalances are often the result of using diuretics; the specific imbalance that develops is related to the class of the drug used and the drug's site of action in the kidneys.

Glossary

The following terms are defined in Appendix A, page 127.

glucocorticoid

mineralocorticoid

renin-angiotensin-aldosterone
mechanism

sympathetic response

Study questions

To evaluate your understanding of this chapter, answer the following questions in the space provided; then compare your responses with the correct answers in Appendix B, page 134.

1. What is the most common acid-base imbalance that occurs in renal failure?

   _____

   _____

2. For what signs and symptoms would the nurse monitor when the patient experiences a fluid volume overload? _____

   _____

3. In a patient with CHF, the imbalances that occur can result from what circumstances? _____

   _____

4. What is the most common acid-base imbalance for the patient with respiratory insufficiency? _____

   _____

5. What imbalance usually develops 3 to 5 days after a major burn injury?

   _____

   _____

6. For the patient with DKA experiencing metabolic acidosis, why should the nurse administer parenteral K slowly? _____

   _____

7. What is HNKS characterized by? _____

   _____

8. In SIADH, from what do fluid imbalances result? _____

   _____

   _____

Study questions *(continued)*

9. What happens when an intestinal obstruction occurs? _____

_____

_____

10. What are the most common causes of fluid and electrolyte imbalances?

_____

_____

11. What acid-base imbalance would the nurse anticipate if the patient experi
ences prolonged vomiting? _____

_____

12. What imbalance is most commonly seen with diuretic use? _____

_____

_____

Appendices

A: Glossary

Acid – substance that is an H ion donor

Acidosis – abnormal state resulting from the gain of H ion donors or H ion acceptors

Aldosterone – adrenocortical hormone that regulates Na and K balance

Alkalosis – abnormal state resulting from the loss of H ion donors or H ion acceptors

Anuria – no urine output

Arrhythmia – abnormal cardiac rhythm usually caused by alterations in normal cardiac conduction

Asterixis – hand-flapping tremor commonly accompanying metabolic disorders

Base – substance that is an H ion acceptor

Body fluid – fluid composed of water and solutes and contained in the ICF and ECF compartments

Buffer – substance that minimizes pH changes by absorbing hydrogen ions when a base is added to the system and releasing hydrogen ions when an acid is added

Chvostek's sign – physical assessment test for hypocalcemia involving lightly tapping the facial nerve (located on the upper cheek below the zygomatic bone); abnormal spasm of facial muscles points to hypocalcemia

Circumoral paresthesia – numbness and tingling around the lips and mouth

Colloid – solution composed of serum proteins and albumin in plasma

Crystalloid – solution composed of water and solutes (primarily electrolytes) administered for hydration

Electrolyte – element or compound that, when melted or dissolved in water or another solvent, dissociates into ions that carry an electrical charge

Extracellular dehydration — water deficit in the extracellular compartment

Gastrostomy — surgically created opening into the stomach through the abdominal wall for insertion of a feeding tube

Glucocorticoid — steroid secreted from the adrenal cortex that is involved with the postoperative stress response

Hydrostatic pressure — pressure exerted by a liquid

Hypertonic — having a higher solute concentration than another solution

Hyperventilation — rapid respiratory rate commonly associated with anxiety

Hypotonic — having a lower solute concentration than another solution

Hypoventilation — abnormally reduced respiratory rate and depth

Intracellular dehydration — water deficit in the intracellular compartment

Ion — solute with a positive or negative electrical charge; positively charged ions are known as cations, and negatively charged ions are known as anions

Isotonic — having the same solute concentration as another solution, such as normal body fluids

Kussmaul respirations — abnormally deep, rapid respirations resulting from air hunger; a compensatory mechanism characteristic of diabetic acidosis

Mineralocorticoid — substance secreted from the adrenal cortex, such as aldosterone, that causes Na retention in renal tubules

Myoneural junction — area of contact between the ends of a large myelinated nerve fiber and a skeletal muscle fiber

Oliguria — daily urine output between 50 to 400 ml

Osmolality — osmotic pressure of a solution expressed in milliosmols per kilogram of solution

Osmolarity — the osmotic pressure of a solution expressed in milliosmols per liter of solution

Osmoreceptor cells — specialized cells in the hypothalamus that respond to serum osmolality and trigger the thirst sensation

Parenteral fluid—solution administered intravenously

Polyuria—urine output greater than fluid intake

Renin-angiotensin-aldosterone mechanism—renal mechanism that increases blood pressure by causing peripheral vasoconstriction and Na and water retention

Specific gravity—weight of a substance in relation to the weight of an equal volume of water; normal urine specific gravity ranges from 1.003 to 1.030; water is considered to have a specific gravity of 1.000

Sympathetic response—reaction by a part of the autonomic nervous system that increases the heart rate and causes peripheral vasoconstriction

Tetany—condition indicating abnormal calcium metabolism characterized by cramps, convulsions, muscle twitching, and sharp wrist and ankle joint flexion

Third space—an abnormal compartment created by a change in the normal cellular membrane caused by trauma, edema, or manipulation, for example, abscess, ascites, or burns

Thyrotoxicosis—life-threatening disorder associated with pronounced hyperthyroidism; also known as Graves' disease

Transcellular water—highly specialized fluid found in specific areas, such as gastric juices and cerebrospinal fluid

Trousseau's sign—physical assessment test for hypocalcemia involving applying a blood pressure cuff to the upper arm and inflating it to a pressure 20 mm Hg above the patient's systolic blood pressure; carpal spasm points to hypocalcemia

B: Answers to Study Questions

CHAPTER 1

1. Body fluid is considered an isotonic solution.

2. Body water is divided into the intracellular and extracellular fluid compartments.

3. Electrolytes refer to solutes that generate an electrical charge when dissolved in water.

4. Potassium is the major intracellular cation; sodium is the major extracellular cation.

5. The sodium-potassium pump moves sodium from the cells to the ECF.

6. pH refers to the acidity or alkalinity of a solution, which is determined by the hydrogen ion concentration.

7. The normal arterial blood pH ranges from 7.35 to 7.45.

CHAPTER 2

1. A 1-lb weight gain is equivalent to a fluid gain of 500 ml.

2. The primary source of water intake is through ingested liquids, accounting for approximately 1,500 ml per day.

3. The normal range for serum osmolality is 280 to 295 mOsm/liter.

4. An increase in serum osmolality results in increased secretion of ADH from the posterior pituitary gland, promoting water reabsorption in the renal tubules; thus, less urine is excreted.

5. The amount of urine produced each day by the kidneys is influenced by aldosterone and ADH levels.

CHAPTER 3

1. Na level is controlled by the feedback loop in which aldosterone secretion by the adrenal cortex stimulates the renal tubules to reabsorb Na.

2. Major functions of K include maintaining cell electroneutrality and cell osmolality; directly affecting cardiac muscle contraction and electrical conductivity; aiding neuromuscular transmission of nerve impulses; and playing a major role in acid-base balance.

3. K and Na have a reciprocal relationship; aldosterone secretion results in renal Na reabsorption and renal K excretion. Because potassium ions are exchanged for hydrogen ions, in acid-base balance, a decrease in potassium excretion accompanies an increase in hydrogen ion excretion.

4. Decreased chloride losses (for example, in vomiting) result in an increased bicarbonate level to balance anions and cations in the ECF.

5. When serum becomes alkaline, more calcium binds to protein; thus, symptoms of hypocalcemia usually occur during alkalosis.

6. Functions of Mg include activating intracellular enzymes and acting in carbohydrate and protein metabolism; acting on the myoneural junction, affecting neuromuscular irritability and contractility of cardiac and skeletal muscle; affecting peripheral vasodilation; facilitating transport of Na and K across the cell membrane; and influencing intracellular Ca level through its effect on PTH secretion.

CHAPTER 4

1. $PaCO_2$ values indicate the partial pressure of CO_2 in arterial blood and are used to evaluate the respiratory acid-base component.

2. The normal range for HCO_3 values is 22 to 26 mEq/liter. Values greater than 26 mEq/liter indicate metabolic alkalosis; values less than 22 mEq/liter indicate metabolic acidosis.

3. The major extracellular chemical buffers are carbonic acid (H_2CO_3) and sodium bicarbonate ($NaHCO_3$).

4. The lungs are the first line of protection in acid-base regulation.

5. In metabolic acidosis, the lungs compensate by increasing the rate and depth of respirations and greater elimination of CO_2.

6. The kidneys may excrete either acidic or alkaline urine to compensate for excesses. They reabsorb HCO_3 from the renal tubule in a state of acid excess and excrete HCO_3 from the renal tubule in a state of acid deficit. Hydrogen ions combine with phosphates and are excreted as phosphoric acid; H ions combine H with ammonia (NH_3) to form ammonium (NH_4).

CHAPTER 5

1. An ECF volume deficit results from relatively equal losses of Na and water.

2. Clinical manifestations of ECF volume excess include acute weight gain, distended neck veins, polyuria, elevated blood pressure, full bounding pulse, crackles, dyspnea, tachypnea, ascites, and peripheral edema.

3. An ICF volume excess results from a disproportionate gain of water in relation to Na^+ in the ECF.

4. Three key causes of ICF volume excess include I.V. administration of hypotonic solutions, tap water enemas, and replacement of lost body fluids with water only.

5. For the patient with ICF volume deficit, the serum Na level would be greater than 145 mEq/liter.

6. For the patient with a third-space fluid shift, the nurse should monitor and document the following to assess the extent and severity of the third-space shift: pulse rate and rhythm, blood pressure, respiratory rate, fluid intake and output, daily weight, abdominal girth, and urine specific gravity and osmolality.

CHAPTER 6

1. Three key causes of hyponatremia are prolonged diuretic therapy, excessive diaphoresis, and insufficient Na intake; excess water intake also may contribute.

2. The primary treatment for hyponatremia is fluid restriction.

3. Clinical manifestations of hypernatremia include extreme thirst; tachycardia; low-grade fever; dry, sticky tongue and oral mucosa; disorientation; hallucinations; lethargy progressing to coma; hyperactive deep tendon reflexes; seizures; coma; hypertension; oliguria or anuria; and agitation.

4. Approximately 40 mEq of K are excreted in 1 liter of urine under normal circumstances.

5. ECG changes in hypokalemia include ST segment depression, flattened T waves, and U waves present or superimposed on the T waves.

6. K replacement therapy is administered orally or by I.V. infusion slowly as a diluted solution. It is never given through I.V. push or as a bolus medication.

7. Excessive K acts as a myocardial depressant, resulting in a decreased heart rate, decreased cardiac output, and possible cardiac arrest.

8. The nurse must assess the patient for arrhythmias because Ca sensitizes the heart to digitalis and if Ca is administered too rapidly, cardiac arrest may occur.

9. Hypophosphatemia commonly results from decreased intestinal absorption of P.

10. The nurse should teach the patient and family about the dangers of diuretic abuse and its link to hypomagnesemia and also about foods high in Mg, such as green vegetables, nuts, beans, and fruits.

11. ECG changes in hypermagnesemia include widened QRS complex, prolonged PR interval, and elevated T wave.

12. Feeding an infant cow's milk rather than formula or breast milk can cause hyperphosphatemia because of the higher P level in cow's milk.

CHAPTER 7

1. Respiratory acidosis is defined by a low arterial pH and elevated serum CO_2 levels.

2. Nursing interventions are directed at improving oxygenation and ventilation.

3. The body attempts to compensate for respiratory acidosis by increasing the renal reabsorption of HCO_3.

4. For the patient with respiratory alkalosis, ABG findings include $PaCO_2$ levels below 35 mm Hg, arterial pH above 7.45, and normal HCO_3 and PaO_2 levels.

5. The nurse can instruct the patient to breathe slowly and less deeply, and if necessary, the nurse can have the patient breathe into a paper bag to decrease CO_2 loss.

6. The body attempts to compensate for metabolic acidosis through hyperventilation, which results in decreased $PaCO_2$.

7. For the patient with chronic metabolic acidosis, the nurse can provide a diet high in carbohydrates and low in fat, which will decrease metabolic waste products and thus ameliorate acidosis.

8. Four key etiologic reasons for developing metabolic alkalosis are excessive administration or ingestion of HCO_3; excessive loss of H ions from NG suctioning or vomiting; prolonged diuretic therapy, particularly K-wasting diuretics; and $NaHCO_3$ administration during cardiopulmonary resuscitation.

9. ABG findings for the patient with uncompensated metabolic alkalosis include arterial pH greater than 7.45, arterial HCO_3 level greater than 26 mEq/liter, $PaCO_2$ level 35 to 45 mm Hg, base excess positive, and serum CO_2 level greater than 28 mEq/liter.

10. Diagnostic findings commonly seen in metabolic acidosis include an arterial pH of less than 7.35, arterial HCO_3 of less than 22 mEq/liter, normal $PaCO_2$, negative base excess, and a serum CO_2 level of less than 22 mEq/liter.

CHAPTER 8

1. Isotonic fluids have the same osmolality as plasma.

2. Crystalloid solutions are used to provide hydration, provide calories, spare protein from use as a source of energy (D_5W), correct Na and Cl deficits (0.9-percent sodium chloride), replace ECF losses (0.9-percent sodium chloride), and correct acidosis (lactated Ringer's solution).

3. The nurse must check the placement of the NG tube before any feeding.

4. The safest ways of verifying feeding tube placement include X-ray and aspirating gastric contents with a pH of less than 4.0.

5. TPN should be administered slowly, using an infusion pump through a central venous site.

6. Colloids are administered during acute situations to expand intravascular volume and maintain blood pressure.

7. The nurse should assess for signs and symptoms of blood transfusion reaction, such as fever, chills, shortness of breath, headache, and hematuria. If a reaction occurs, the nurse must stop the infusion immediately and infuse normal saline solution to keep the vein open, using a new administration set; take the patient's vital signs; notify the physician; and follow institution policies for further actions.

CHAPTER 9

1. The most common acid-base imbalance that occurs in renal failure is metabolic acidosis.

2. For the patient with a fluid volume overload, the nurse would monitor for edema, bounding pulse, and shortness of breath.

3. Imbalances associated with CHF can result from the heart's failure to pump and to adequately perfuse the tissues, from stimulation of the renin-angiotensin-aldosterone mechanism, or from treatment interventions, such as diuretics.

4. In respiratory insufficiency, the most common acid-base imbalance is respiratory acidosis.

5. An ECF volume excess usually develops 3 to 5 days after a major burn injury.

6. The nurse should administer parenteral K slowly because correction of metabolic acidosis releases K from the cells, thereby increasing the possibility of developing hyperkalemia.

7. HNKS is characterized by hyperglycemia, hyperosmolality, and osmotic diuresis; ketosis and ketonuria do not occur.

8. In SIADH, fluid imbalances result from the continuous and inappropriate secretion of ADH, leading to water retention, which leads to serum hypo-osmolality.

9. When an intestinal obstruction occurs, a large amount of water and electrolytes are secreted into the bowel or peritoneal space, creating a third space.

10. The most common causes of fluid and electrolyte imbalances is GI fluid loss.

11. For the patient with prolonged vomiting, the nurse would anticipate metabolic alkalosis.

12. Hypokalemia is the most commonly seen imbalance with diuretic use.

C: Fluid Balance Checklist

Below is a quick reference checklist to assess a patient's fluid balance status. Remember your priorities are to establish baseline vital signs and weight, then to monitor and record daily vital signs, weight, and fluid intake and output.

ASSESSMENT CHECKLIST	PROBLEMS
Monitor weight	
☐ Loss of 5% or less ☐ Loss of 5% to 10% ☐ Loss of more than 10%	Mild dehydration Moderate dehydration Severe dehydration
☐ Gain of 5% or less ☐ Gain of 5% to 10% ☐ Gain of more than 10%	Mild overhydration Moderate overhydration Severe overhydration
Observe eyes	
☐ Dry conjunctiva ☐ Decreased tearing ☐ Periorbital edema ☐ Sunken eyes ☐ Soft eyeballs	Fluid volume deficit
Observe mouth	
☐ Sticky, dry mucous membranes	Fluid volume deficit Sodium excess
☐ Increased viscosity of saliva	Sodium deficit
Observe lips	
☐ Dry, cracked	Fluid volume deficit
Observe tongue	
☐ Longitudinal furrows	Sodium deficit
Assess cardiovascular system	
☐ Increased pulse rate ☐ Decreased pulse rate ☐ Decreased blood pressure ☐ Narrow pulse pressure	Fluid volume deficit
☐ Bounding pulse ☐ Jugular vein distension	Fluid volume excess
☐ Cardiac arrhythmias	Potassium deficit Magnesium deficit

(continued)

Fluid Balance Checklist *(continued)*

ASSESSMENT CHECKLIST	PROBLEMS
Assess respiratory system	
☐ Moist crackles, rhonchi ☐ Increased respiratory rate ☐ Dyspnea ☐ Pulmonary edema	Fluid volume excess
☐ Shallow, slow breathing	Respiratory alkalosis with or without metabolic acidosis
☐ Deep, rapid breathing	Respiratory acidosis with or without metabolic alkalosis
Assess GI system	
☐ Absent bowel sounds (ileus)	Potassium deficit
☐ Abdominal cramps	Potassium excess
☐ Nausea, vomiting, and diarrhea	Magnesium excess
☐ Nausea, diarrhea	Potassium excess
☐ Nausea, vomiting, and constipation	Calcium excess
Assess renal system	
☐ Oliguria	Sodium deficit or excess Potassium excess
Observe extremities	
☐ Edema of dependent body parts (including sacrum and lower extremities)	Fluid volume excess
Observe skin condition	
☐ Warm	Sodium excess
☐ Cold, clammy	Sodium deficit
☐ Cold ☐ Poor skin turgor	Fluid volume deficit
☐ Warm, moist	Fluid volume excess
☐ Flushing	Magnesium deficit
Assess neurologic condition	
☐ Depressed central nervous system	Fluid volume deficit Electrolyte imbalance
☐ Increased intracranial pressure	Sodium deficit

Fluid Balance Checklist *(continued)*

ASSESSMENT CHECKLIST	PROBLEMS
Assess neurologic condition *(continued)*	
☐ Positive Babinski's sign	Magnesium deficit
☐ Disorientation or confusion	Fluid volume excess Acidosis or alkalosis Electrolyte imbalance
☐ Seizures	Calcium deficit Magnesium deficit
Observe musculoskeletal system	
☐ Muscle weakness	Potassium deficit Calcium excess
☐ Paralysis of flaccid muscles	Potassium excess
☐ Numbness in extremities	Potassium excess
☐ Hypertonicity (physical checks include positive Chvostek's sign, carpopedal spasm, Trousseau's sign)	Metabolic alkalosis Calcium deficit Magnesium deficit
☐ Muscle rigidity	Metabolic alkalosis
Monitor laboratory test results	
☐ Hematocrit elevation	Fluid volume excess or deficit Sodium excess
☐ Protein elevation	None
☐ Protein depletion	Malnutrition Starvation Third-space shifting
☐ Increased urine pH	Metabolic and respiratory alkalosis
☐ Decreased urine pH	Metabolic and respiratory acidosis
☐ Elevated BUN and normal serum creatinine	Fluid volume deficit
Monitor urine specific gravity	
☐ Elevation	Fluid volume deficit
☐ Decrease	Sodium deficit
☐ Red blood cell increase	Sodium excess or deficit Fluid volume overload

D: Standard I.V. Solutions Used for Fluid and Electrolyte Replacement Therapy

PRODUCT	OSMOLARITY	ELECTROLYTES	
		ELEMENT	AMOUNT
Dextrose solutions			
• 2.5%	126 mOsm/liter	N/A	N/A
• 5%	252 mOsm/liter	N/A	N/A
• 10%	505 mOsm/liter	N/A	N/A
• 20%	1,010 mOsm/liter	N/A	N/A
• 50%	2,525 mOsm/liter	N/A	N/A
Saline solutions			
• 0.45%	154 mOsm/liter	Sodium chloride	77 mEq/liter
• 0.9%	308 mOsm/liter	Sodium chloride	154 mEq/liter
• 3%	1,026 mOsm/liter	Sodium chloride	513 mEq/liter
• 5%	1,710 mOsm/liter	Sodium chloride	855 mEq/liter
Dextrose-saline solutions			
• 5% D/0.45 normal saline	406 mOsm/liter	Sodium chloride	77 mEq/liter
• 5% D/0.9 normal saline	559 mOsm/liter	Sodium chloride	154 mEq/liter
Ringer's (plain) solution			
	309 mOsm/liter	Sodium	130 mEq/liter
		Potassium	4 mEq/liter
		Calcium	3 mEq/liter
		Chloride	109 mEq/liter
Lactated Ringer's solution			
	273 mOsm/liter	Sodium	130 mEq/liter
		Potassium	4 mEq/liter
		Calcium	3 mEq/liter
		Chloride	109 mEq/liter
		Lactate	28 mEq/liter
Dextrose			
In lactated Ringer's solution			
• 2.5%	265 mOsm/liter		
• 5%	525 mOsm/liter	(see "Lactated Ringer's solution" above)	(see "Lactated Ringer's solution" above)
• 10%	775 mOsm/liter		
In Ringer's (plain) solution	N/A	(see "Ringer's [plain] solution" above)	(see "Ringer's [plain] solution" above)
• 2.5%	562 mOsm/liter		
• 5%	N/A		
• 10%			

CALORIES PER LITER AND INDICATIONS	PRECAUTIONS AND NURSING IMPLICATIONS
80 to 1,700 calories. Maintains water balance and corrects imbalance. Supplies calories as carbohydrates.	Electrolyte-free solutions may cause peripheral circulatory collapse and anuria in patients with sodium deficiency. May aggravate hypokalemia and irritate veins. Do not administer with blood. Electrolyte-free solution increases body fluid loss.
No calories. Fluid replacement, dehydration, sodium depletion. Low-salt syndrome (hyponatremia).	Use chloride solution with caution in edematous patients with heart, renal, or hepatic disease. Administer slowly.
170 calories. Fluid replacement, caloric feeding, dehydration, sodium depletion.	Use chloride solution with caution in patients with compromised cardiovascular or pulmonary status. Continually assess for crackles, edema, and skin turgor.
No calories. Dehydration, sodium depletion, replacement of GI loss.	Assess laboratory values for correction of electrolyte imbalance. Continually assess for signs and symptoms of electrolyte imbalances.
9 calories. Replacement of surgical and GI loss, dehydration, sodium depletion, acidosis, diarrhea, and burns.	Check urine output before infusing potassium. Continually assess for electrolyte or fluid imbalance; check laboratory values as well as signs and symptoms specific to imbalance. Assess for edema and crackles.
89 to 349 calories. Supplies calories as carbohydrates.	Do not infuse with blood. Assess patient for greater caloric need.

(continued)

Standard I.V. Solutions Used for Fluid and Electrolyte Replacement Therapy *(continued)*

PRODUCT	OSMOLARITY	ELECTROLYTES	
		ELEMENT	AMOUNT
Dextran 40 and 70			
Dextran 40			
● 10% injection with 5% dextrose	252 mOsm/liter	Sodium	77 mEq/500 ml
● 10% injection with normal saline solution	308 mOsm/liter	Chloride	77 mEq/500 ml
Dextran 70			
● 6% injection with 5% dextrose	N/A	N/A	N/A
● 6% injection with normal saline solution	N/A	N/A	N/A
Mannitol			
● 5% in 0.45 normal saline	275 mOsm/liter	Sodium	77 mEq/liter
● 10% in 0.45 normal saline	550 mOsm/liter	Chloride	
● 20% in 0.45 normal saline	1100 mOsm/liter	77 mEq/liter	

CALORIES PER LITER AND INDICATIONS	PRECAUTIONS AND NURSING IMPLICATIONS
Both, 170 calories. For shock when blood products are not available. Increases blood volume, venous return, cardiac output; decreases blood viscosity and peripheral venous resistance; reduces aggregation of erythrocytes and other blood elements. Prophylaxis against venous thrombosis and thromboembolism. Inhibits vascular stasis and platelet adhesiveness. Priming solution for extracorporeal circulation, decreases destruction of erythrocytes and platelets, reduces intravascular hemagglutination, and reduces danger of serum hepatitis and transfusion reactions.	Watch for allergic reactions (such as mild urticaria) and stop infusion immediately (these colloid hypertonic solutions attract water from the extravascular space and can cause fluid overload). Infuse cautiously in dehydrated patients, in whom additional fluid replacement will be needed. May prolong bleeding time and depress platelet function; may decrease renal and liver function. Can alter the following laboratory values: blood glucose, bilirubin, and total protein values; blood typing; cross matching; and tests with acids.
No calories. Test for renal function (oliguria from tubular necrosis). Diuretic therapy for intoxications, edema, and ascites.	Do not give to patients with impaired renal function who fail to respond to the test dose, with severe congestive heart failure, or with metabolic edema and head injuries. Low room temperature may cause crystallization. Use blood filter set to prevent infusion of mannitol crystals.

E: Food and Fluid Sources of Major Electrolytes

ELECTROLYTE	MAJOR FOOD SOURCES	MAJOR FUNCTIONS
CALCIUM	Bonemeal, cheese, milk, molasses, yogurt, whole grains, nuts, legumes, leafy vegetables	Blood clotting, bone and tooth formation, cardiac rhythm regulation, cell membrane structure and function, muscle growth and contraction, nerve impulse transmission
CHLORIDE	Fruits, vegetables, table salt	Maintenance of fluid, electrolyte, acid-base, and osmotic pressure balance
MAGNESIUM	Green leafy vegetables, nuts, seafood, cocoa, whole grains	Acid-base balance, calcium and phosphorus metabolism in bones, muscle relaxation, cellular respiration, nerve impulse transmission, cardiac muscle function and maintenance
PHOSPHORUS	Eggs, fish, grains, meats, poultry, yellow cheese, milk, milk products	Bone and tooth formation, cell growth and repair, energy production, kidney function, metabolism (carbohydrates, fats, proteins), myocardial contraction, nerve and muscle activity, acid-base balance
POTASSIUM	Seafood, molasses, bananas, peaches, peanuts, raisins	Heartbeat, muscle contraction, nerve impulse transmission, fluid distribution and osmotic pressure balance, acid-base balance
SODIUM	Seafood, cheese, milk, salt	Extracellular fluid, osmotic pressure balance, muscle contraction, acid-base and water balance, cell permeability, muscle function, nerve impulse transmission

F: Arterial Blood Gas Findings and Interpretations

To help determine a patient's acid-base status, use the chart below. Keep in mind that your hospital's laboratory may use values that differ slightly from those shown here.

pH	Paco$_2$	HCO$_3^-$	IMPLICATION	CAUSE
Below 7.35	Normal	Below 22	Metabolic acidosis— uncompensated	Acid gain or base loss (causing base deficit)
Below 7.35	Below 35	Below 22	Metabolic acidosis— partially compensated	Acid gain or base loss (causing base deficit)
Normal or near normal	Below 35	Below 22	Metabolic acidosis— compensated	Acid gain or base loss (causing base deficit)
Below 7.35	Above 45	Normal	Respiratory acidosis— uncompensated	Hypoventilation
Below 7.35	Above 45	Above 26	Respiratory acidosis— partially compensated	Hypoventilation
Normal or near normal	Above 45	Above 26	Respiratory acidosis— compensated	Hypoventilation
Above 7.45	Normal	Above 26	Metabolic alkalosis— uncompensated	Base gain or acid loss (causing base excess)
Above 7.45	Above 45	Above 26	Metabolic alkalosis— partially compensated	Base gain or acid loss (causing base excess)
Normal or near normal	Above 45	Above 26	Metabolic alkalosis— compensated	Base gain or acid loss (causing base excess)
Above 7.45	Below 35	Normal	Respiratory alkalosis— uncompensated	Hyperventilation
Above 7.45	Below 35	Below 22	Respiratory alkalosis— partially compensated	Hyperventilation
Normal or near normal	Below 35	Below 22	Respiratory alkalosis— compensated	Hyperventilation
Below 7.35	Above 45	Below 22	Combined respiratory acidosis and metabolic acidosis	Hypoventilation, plus acid gain or base loss
Above 7.45	Below 35	Above 26	Combined respiratory alkalosis and metabolic alkalosis	Hyperventilation, plus base gain or acid loss

(continued)

Arterial Blood Gas Findings and Interpretations (continued)

pH	Paco₂	HCO₃⁻	IMPLICATION	CAUSE
Variable (depends on which disorder is more severe)	Above 45	Above 26	Mixed respiratory acidosis and metabolic alkalosis	Hypoventilation, plus base gain or acid loss
Variable (depends on which disorder is more severe)	Below 35	Below 22	Mixed respiratory alkalosis and metabolic acidosis	Hyperventilation, plus acid gain or base loss

G: Blood Component Therapy

All blood component products are extracted from whole blood, but because each has different characteristics, some components treat certain hematologic disorders better than others. The doctor will choose a blood component product based on how well it will treat your patient's condition. For example, if your patient needs volume replenishment quickly, he or she will receive a volume expander. If his or her blood is not clotting properly, he or she will receive a product with clotting factors. The table below reviews blood component products and their uses.

TYPE	CONTENTS	USES	NURSING CONSIDERATIONS
Whole blood	• Red blood cells (RBCs), white blood cells (WBCs), platelets, plasma, and plasma clotting factors	• To restore blood volume and to replenish oxygen-carrying capacity in a patient with massive hemorrhage	• Administer through a large-gauge needle or catheter over 2 to 4 hours, or as prescribed.
Packed cells	• RBCs and 20% plasma • Less sodium and potassium than whole blood	• To replenish blood's oxygen-carrying capacity while minimizing risk of fluid overload in patients with severe anemia, slow blood loss, or congestive heart failure	• Administer over 2 to 4 hours. • Do not use for anemic conditions correctable by nutrition or drug therapy.
Washed cells	• RBCs and 20% plasma • Fewer WBCs and platelets than packed cells	• To replenish blood's oxygen-carrying capacity in patients previously sensitized by transfusions	• Infuse over 1½ to 4 hours.
Granulocytes	• WBCs and 20% plasma	• To treat life-threatening granulocytopenia ($< 500/mm^3$)	• Administer rapidly. • Expect the patient to develop fever, chills, hypertension, or disorientation during transfusion; these are considered transfusion reactions.
Plasma (fresh frozen)	• Clotting factors II, III, V, VII, IX, X, and XIII; fibrinogen; prothrombin; albumin; and globulins	• To treat patients with clotting factor deficiencies (the only treatment for factor V deficiency) • To expand volume	• Administer at a rate of 10 ml/minute. • Use within 6 hours of thawing.

(continued)

Blood Component Therapy *(continued)*

TYPE	CONTENTS	USES	NURSING CONSIDERATIONS
Platelets	• Platelets, WBCs, and plasma	• To correct low platelet counts ($<10,000/mm^3$)	• Administer one unit over 10 minutes.
Cryoprecipitate	• Factors VIII and XIII and fibrinogen	• To replace clotting factors in patients with disseminated intravascular coagulation, hemophilia A, von Willebrand's disease, fibrinogen deficiency, or factor XIII deficiency	• Administer rapidly immediately after thawing to ensure factor activation.
Albumin (5% and 25%)	• 5% and 25% albumin from plasma	• To replace volume in patients suffering from shock, burns, hypoproteinemia, or hypoalbuminemia	• Administer 1 ml/ minute or, if the patient is in shock, administer rapidly. • May administer with dextrose 5% in water.
Plasma protein fraction	• 5% albumin and globulin solution in normal saline solution	• To expand volume in patients with burns, hemorrhage, or hypoproteinemia	• Administer 1 ml/ minute. • Risk of hepatitis or sensitization is low.

Selected References

Blevis, L.S., and Ward, G.S. "Diabetes Insipidus," *Critical Care Medicine* 20(1):69-79, 1992.

Boyle, M.A., and Zyle, G. *Personal Nutrition*, 2nd ed. New York: West Publishing Co., 1992.

Burchard, K.W., et al. "Hypocalcemia During Sepsis: Relationship to Resuscitation and Hemodynamics," *Archives of Surgery* 127(3):265-272, March 1992.

Chen, T.Y. "Life Threatening Hyperkalemia in an Elderly Patient Receiving Captopril, Furosemide and Potassium Supplements," *Drug Safety* 7(2):159-161, 1992.

Charles, P. "Calcium Absorption and Calcium Bioavailability," *Journal of Internal Medicine* 231:161-168, 1992.

Dunezt, P.S. "If Your Med/Surg Patient Is on Dialysis, *RN.* 46-53, September 1992.

Hamill, R.J., et al. "Efficacy and Safety of Potassium Infusion Therapy in Hypokalemic Critically-Ill Patients," *Critical Care Medicine* 19(5):694-699, 1991.

Hamilton, E.M., et al., *Nutrition: Concept and Controversy*, 5th ed. New York: West Publishing Co., 1991.

Harkema, J.M., and Chaudry, I.H. "Magnesium-Adenosine Triphosphate in the Treatment of Shock, Ischemia and Sepsis," *Critical Care Medicine* 20(2):263-273, 1992.

Heink, N.R. "Fluid Resuscitation and the Role of Exchange Transfusion on Pediatric Burn Shock," *Critical Care Nurse* 12(7):50-56, October, 1992.

Innerarity, S.A. "Electrolyte Emergencies in the Critically Ill Renal Patient," *Critical Care Nursing Clinics of North America* 2(1):89-99, March 1990.

Johnson, K., and Kligman, E.W. "Preventative Nutrition: Disease Specific Dietary Interventions for Older Adults," *Geriatrics* 47(11):39-49, 1992.

Keyes, J. *Fluid, Electrolyte, and Acid-Base Regulation: Physiology & Pathophysiology.* Boston: Jones & Bartlett Publishers, Inc., 1985.

Khilnani, P. "Electrolyte Abnormalities in Critically-Ill Children," *Critical Care Medicine* 20(2):241-250, 1992.

Kinney, M.R., et al. *AACN's Clinical Reference for Critical Care Nursing*, 3rd ed. New York: Mosby, Inc., 1993.

Koch, S.M., and Taylor, R.W. "Chloride Ion in Intensive Care Medicine," *Critical Care Medicine* 20(2):227-240, 1992.

Metheny, N. *Fluid and Electrolyte Balance*, 2nd ed. Philadelphia: J.B. Lippincott Co., 1992.

Millene, T.A., et al. "Is Hypomagnesemia Arrhythogenic," *Critical Cardiology* 15(2):103-108, February 1992.

Mizock, B.A., and Falk, J.L. "Lactic Acidosis in Critical Illness," *Critical Care Medicine* 20(1):80-93, 1992.

Norris, M.K. "Assessing Elevated Potassium Values," *Nursing* 21(1):31, January 1991.

Oh, M.S., and Carroll, H.J. "Disorders of Sodium Metabolism: Hypernatremia and Hyponatremia," *Critical Care Medicine* 20(1):94-103. 1992.

Plumer, A. *Principles and Practice of Intravenous Therapy*, 4th ed. Glenview, Ill.: Scott, Foresman & Co., 1987.

Porterfield, L.M. "Potassium Replacement" *Advancing Clinical Care* 5(6):18, November-December 1990.

Sieber, F.E., and Traiptman, R.J. "Special Issues: Glucose and the Brain," *Critical Care Medicine* 20(1):104-114, 1992.

Restuccio, A. "Fatal Hyperkalemia from a Salt Substitute," *American Journal of Emergency Medicine* 10(2):171-173, 1992.

Stark, J. "Renal System," in *Core Curriculum for Critical Care Nursing*, edited by Alspach, J.G. Philadelphia: W.B. Saunders Co., 1991.

Stroot, V.R., et al. *Fluids & Electrolytes*, 3rd ed. Philadelphia: F.A. Davis Co., 1984.

Toss, G. "Effects of Calcium Intake vs. Other Life-Style Factors on Bone Mass," *Journal of Internal Medicine* 231:181-186, 1992.

Weldy, N. *Body Fluids and Electrolytes: A Programmed Presentation*, 6th ed. St. Louis: Mosby, Inc., 1992.

Woolf, P.D. "Hormonal Responses to Trauma," *Critical Care Medicine* 20(2):216-226, 1992.

Zaloga, G.P. "Hypocalcemia in Critically-Ill Patients," *Critical Care Medicine* 20(2):251-262, 1992.

Index

---

i refers to an illustration; t, to a table

Notes

Notes